Weaver & Koehler's

PROGRAMMED MATHEMATICS
OF
DRUGS AND SOLUTIONS

Weaver & Koehler's

PROGRAMMED MATHEMATICS

OF

DRUGS AND SOLUTIONS

FIFTH EDITION

VIRGINIA POOLE ARCANGELO, RN, PhD
Assistant Professor
Department of Nursing
College of Allied Health Sciences
Thomas Jefferson University
Philadelphia, Pennsylvania

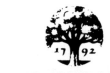

J.B. LIPPINCOTT COMPANY
Philadelphia
New York   London   Hagerstown

Acquiring Editor: Ellen Campbell
Production Supervisor: Robert D. Bartleson
Production: Publishers' WorkGroup
Compositor: Bucks County Type & Design
Printer/Binder: R. R. Donnelley & Sons Company

5th Edition

6 5 4 3 2 1

Library of Congress Cataloging-in-Publication Data

Arcangelo, Virginia Poole.
    Weaver & Koehler's programmed mathematics of drugs and solutions.
—5th ed. / Virginia Poole Arcangelo.
      p. cm.
    Rev. ed. of: Programmed mathematics of drugs and solutions / Mabel E. Weaver, Vera J. Koehler ; revising author, Virginia Poole Arcangelo. 1984 revision. c1984.
    ISBN 0-397-54918-0 (pbk.)
    1. Pharmaceutical arithmetic—Programmed instruction.   I. Weaver, Mabel E.   II. Koehler, Vera J.   III. Weaver, Mabel E.   Programmed mathematics of drugs and solutions.   IV. Title.   V. Title: Weaver and Koehler's programmed mathematics of drugs and solutions.
VI. Title: Programmed mathematics of drugs and solutions.
    [DNLM: 1. Mathematics—nurses' instruction.   2. Mathematics-
-programmed instruction.   3. Pharmacy—nurses' instruction.
4. Pharmacy—programmed instruction.   QV 18 A668w]
RS57.A73   1992
615'.1'01513—dc20
DNLM/DLC   91–19708
for Library of Congress   CIP

The author and the publisher would like to acknowledge the contributions of Mabel E. Weaver, RN, MS, Professor Emeritus, and Vera J. Koehler, RN, MN, Professor Emeritus, both of the Division of Nursing at California State University, Sacramento, to the original edition of this text and its subsequent revisions.

PREFACE

This book is designed to be both a self-paced introductory program to the mathematics of drugs and solutions and a refresher for knowledge previously learned. It provides a review of basic arithmetic and the application of those concepts to drugs and solutions. The book can be helpful to student nurses and practicing nurses alike.

The reader's knowledge is tested at various points. A pretest is included to provide guidelines to areas of weakness in basic arithmetic. Numerous practice problems throughout the book provide an immediate measure of the reader's understanding of the concepts. A comprehensive examination is included at the end of the book.

This fifth edition includes a chapter of basic arithmetic review, for those who need a refresher in that area. Every drug name and dosage has been reviewed for current use. The chapter on intravenous medications has been expanded to include calculations of drips based on dosages ordered.

VIRGINIA POOLE ARCANGELO, RN, PhD

TO THE READER

One important part of nursing practice is the correct administration of drugs and solutions to patients. In order to provide a person with the correct dosage of medication, the nurse may need to do some mathematical calculations, for the drug available may be stated in a different system of measurement or may be more or less than the amount that has been ordered. The goal of this book is to enable you to solve such problems.

To do this, mathematical concepts are presented in a practical way within the text. These concepts are then applied to the preparation of drugs and solutions. It is your responsibility to learn the mathematical skills necessary to administer medications accurately.

The names of drugs found in the problems and examples are currently used in practice. A section on proper selection and use of syringes is included.

This is a programmed textbook. It may be different from books you have used in the past in that the text is incomplete and broken down into small units called "frames." You will complete the text by filling in words or phrases or by answering the questions. The answers can be written in the frames. Check each answer as soon as you have written it by comparing it with the correct answer, which is found to the right of the frame you have just read. As you work through the program, use a strip of paper to cover the answer column. You need not be concerned if you make a mistake. The important thing is to go back and find your error and correct it.

This text will assist you in building on your mathematical skills and enable you to apply them to the clinical setting. Good luck.

CONTENTS

COMMON ABBREVIATIONS

$\overline{aa}$	of each
ac	before meals
AD	right ear
ad lib	as desired
AU	both ears
AS	left ear
b.i.d.	twice a day
$\overline{c}$	with
D/C	discontinue
dr. (ʒ)	dram
elix.	elixir
ext.	extract
Fl.	fluid
g (or gm)	gram
gr	grain
gtt	drop
H.	hour
h.s.	hour of sleep (bedtime)
IM	intramuscular
IV	intravenous
kg	kilogram

KVO	keep vein open
l (L)	liter
M.	minim
μg (or mcg)	microgram
mg	milligram
ml	milliliter
mEq	milliequivalent
NPO	nothing by mouth
OD	right eye
os	mouth
OS	left eye
OU	both eyes
oz (ʒ)	ounce
pc	after meals
per	by
p.o.	by mouth
prn	as needed
q	every
q.d.	every day
q.i.d.	four times a day
q.o.d.	every other day
q.s.	sufficient quantity
s	without
SC	subcutaneous
Sig.	write on label
SL	sublingual
Sol.	solution
ss	one-half
stat	right away
t.i.d.	three times a day
U	unit

TABLE OF EQUIVALENTS

LIQUID MEASUREMENTS

1,000 cc* = 32 fluid ounces = 1 quart

500 cc = 16 fluid ounces = 1 pint

30 cc = 1 ounce = 2 tablespoonfuls

15 cc = 4 fluidrams = 1 tablespoonful

5 cc = 1 fluidram = 1 teaspoonful

1 cc = 15 or 16 minims

0.06 cc = 1 minim = 1 drop

*cc and ml can be used interchangeably (1 cc = 1 ml)

WEIGHTS

1 kg = 2.2 pounds

30 g = 1 ounce

15 g = 4 drams

4 g = grains 60 = 1 dram ($\mathfrak{Z}$)

1 g = grains 15

300 mg = grains 5

200 mg = grains 3

60 mg = grain 1

30 mg = grain $\frac{1}{2}$

10 mg = grain $\frac{1}{6}$

6 mg = grain $\frac{1}{10}$

1 mg = grain $\frac{1}{60}$

0.6 mg = grain $\frac{1}{100}$

0.5 mg = grain $\frac{1}{120}$

0.4 mg = grain $\frac{1}{150}$

0.3 mg = grain $\frac{1}{200}$

0.2 mg = grain $\frac{1}{300}$

0.1 mg = grain $\frac{1}{600}$

LENGTH

2.54 cm = 1 inch

1 cm = 0.39 inch

TEMPERATURE CONVERSIONS

$$°F = \frac{9}{5} °C + 32°$$

$$°C = \frac{5}{9} (°F - 32°)$$

GLOSSARY

Ampule—small glass container for solutions; usually used for one dose then discarded.

Compatible—able to mix with another substance without causing a harmful reaction.

Concentration—content of contained substance in solution.

Dilute—to make less concentrated.

Diluent—agent used to make substance less concentrated.

Electrolyte—compound that separates into charged particles when dissolved in water.

Equivalent—equal in value.

Generic—name of drug that identifies it by other than its trade name.

Hyperalimentation—method for providing total caloric needs intravenously for the undernourished individual.

Hypertonic—greater concentration than that of a solution to which it is compared.

Hypodermic—inserted under the skin.

Hypotonic—lesser concentration than that of a solution to which it is compared.

Isotonic—same concentration as that of a solution to which it is compared.

Nomogram—representation by graph, diagram, or chart of relationship between values.

Parenteral—not through the alimentary canal; i.e., subcutaneous, intramuscular, or intravenous.

Precipitate—deposit separated from a solution.

Proprietary—any chemical or drug used in the treatment of disease if protected against free competition by patent or copyright.

Ratio—relation between two similar things.

Saturated—holding all that can be absorbed.

Solute—substance dissolved in solution.

Solvent—liquid holding another substance in solution.

Stock solution—that substance available.

Unit—specifically defined amount of anything subject to measurement.

U.S.P.—United States Pharmacopeia—a legally recognized compendium of standards for drugs.

PRETEST

This pretest is designed to help you assess your knowledge of and ability to work with fractions and decimals. As you proceed through the programmed text, you will need to apply this knowledge in the calculations to arrive at the proper dosage of medication to administer to your patient.

FRACTIONS

A. Add the following and reduce all fractions to lowest terms:

1. $\frac{2}{3} + \frac{4}{5} =$

2. $\frac{1}{3} + \frac{1}{2} + \frac{5}{6} =$

3. $5\frac{1}{2} + 1\frac{1}{3} + 4\frac{1}{4} =$

4. $1\frac{3}{4} + 5\frac{1}{2} + 11\frac{1}{16} =$

5. $\frac{3}{5} + \frac{4}{9} + \frac{7}{30} =$

B. Subtract the following and reduce all fractions to lowest terms:

1. $\frac{5}{8} - \frac{1}{3} =$

2. $2\frac{2}{3} - 1\frac{3}{4} =$

3. $110\frac{3}{33} - 35\frac{2}{3} =$

4. $5\frac{3}{8} - 2\frac{1}{6} =$

5. $6\frac{4}{5} - 2\frac{2}{3} =$

C. Multiply the following and reduce all fractions to lowest terms:

1. $8 \times \frac{3}{4} =$

2. $\frac{11}{12} \times \frac{4}{5} \times 6\frac{1}{4} =$

3. $6\frac{6}{11} \times 7\frac{1}{3} =$

4. $36 \times \frac{5}{6} \times \frac{3}{8} =$

5. $6\frac{1}{4} \times 4 \times 3\frac{2}{5} =$

D. Divide the following and reduce all fractions to lowest terms:

1. $16 \div \frac{4}{5} =$

2. $8\frac{1}{8} \div \frac{3}{4} =$

3. $8\frac{1}{2} \div \frac{9}{16} \div 8 =$

4. $3\frac{1}{7} \div 1\frac{7}{15} \div 2\frac{2}{7} =$

5. $50\frac{4}{5} \div 1\frac{2}{3} =$

DECIMALS

A. Add the following:

1. 2.8 + 3.4 + 6.0 =

2. 21.35 + 7.06 + 0.03 =

3. 0.002 + 31.6 + 8.6 + 2.23 =

4. 1.653 + 21 + 6.3 + 8.22 =

5. 200.62 + 9.4 + 0.003 + 20.1 =

B. Subtract the following:

1. 10.392 – 8.34 =

2. 20.432 – 16.66 =

3. 10.2 – 4.819 =

4. 11.6 – 5.078 =

5. 25.635 – 20.1 =

C. Multiply the following:

    1. 8.2 × 24.3 =

    2. 2.65 × 0.03 =

    3. 4.753 × 2.564 =

    4. 1.75 × 0.002 =

    5. 10.35 × 0.41 =

D. Divide the following:

    1. 20.3 ÷ 15 =

    2. 50 ÷ 2.5 =

    3. 65 ÷ 2.5 =

    4. 80 ÷ 0.55 =

    5. 2.1 ÷ 0.07 =

PROPORTIONS

Solve for x:

1. $\dfrac{4}{5} = \dfrac{x}{30}$

2. $\dfrac{13}{20} = \dfrac{x}{5}$

3. $\dfrac{5}{6} = \dfrac{8}{x}$

4. $\dfrac{1}{200} = \dfrac{x}{50}$

ANSWERS TO PROBLEMS ON PAGE 1
ADDING FRACTIONS (A)

1. $\frac{10}{15} + \frac{12}{15} = 1\frac{7}{15}$

2. $\frac{2}{6} + \frac{3}{6} + \frac{5}{6} = \frac{10}{6} = 1\frac{4}{6} = 1\frac{2}{3}$

3. $5\frac{6}{12} + 1\frac{4}{12} + 4\frac{3}{12} = 10\frac{13}{12} = 11\frac{1}{12}$

4. $1\frac{12}{16} + 5\frac{8}{16} + 11\frac{1}{16} = 17\frac{21}{16} = 18\frac{5}{16}$

5. $\frac{54}{90} + \frac{40}{90} + \frac{21}{90} = \frac{115}{90} = 1\frac{25}{90} = 1\frac{5}{18}$

ANSWERS TO PROBLEMS ON PAGE 1
SUBTRACTING FRACTIONS (B)

1. $\frac{15}{24} - \frac{8}{24} = \frac{7}{24}$

2. $2\frac{8}{12} - 1\frac{9}{12} = \frac{32}{12} - \frac{21}{12} = \frac{11}{12}$

3. $110\frac{3}{33} - 35\frac{22}{33} = 109\frac{36}{33} - 35\frac{22}{33} = 74\frac{14}{33}$

4. $5\frac{9}{24} - 2\frac{4}{24} = 3\frac{5}{24}$

5. $6\frac{12}{15} - 2\frac{10}{15} = 4\frac{2}{15}$

ANSWERS TO PROBLEMS ON PAGE 2
MULTIPLYING FRACTIONS (C)

1. $\frac{8}{1} \times \frac{3}{4} \times \frac{24}{4} = 6$

2. $\frac{11}{12} \times \frac{4}{5} \times \frac{25}{4} = \frac{1100}{240} = 4\frac{7}{12}$

3. $\frac{72}{11} \times \frac{22}{3} = \frac{1584}{33} = 48$

4. $\frac{36}{1} \times \frac{5}{6} \times \frac{3}{8} = \frac{540}{48} = 11\frac{1}{4}$

5. $\frac{25}{4} \times \frac{4}{1} \times \frac{17}{5} = \frac{1700}{20} = 85$

ANSWERS TO PROBLEMS ON PAGE 2

DIVIDING FRACTIONS (D)

1. $\frac{16}{1} \times \frac{5}{4} = \frac{80}{4} = 20$

2. $\frac{65}{8} \times \frac{4}{3} = \frac{260}{24} = 10\frac{5}{6}$

3. $\frac{17}{2} \times \frac{16}{9} \times \frac{1}{8} = \frac{272}{144} = 1\frac{8}{9}$

4. $\frac{22}{7} \times \frac{15}{22} \times \frac{7}{16} = \frac{2310}{2464} = \frac{15}{16}$

5. $\frac{254}{5} \times \frac{3}{5} = \frac{762}{25} = 30\frac{12}{25}$

ANSWERS TO PROBLEMS ON PAGE 2

ADDING DECIMALS (A)

1. 12.2

2. 28.44

3. 42.432

4. 37.173

5. 230.123

ANSWERS TO PROBLEMS ON PAGE 2

SUBTRACTING DECIMALS (B)

1. 2.052

2. 3.772

3. 5.381

4. 6.522

5. 5.535

ANSWERS TO PROBLEMS ON PAGE 3
MULTIPLYING DECIMALS (C)

1. 199.26
2. 0.0795
3. 12.186692
4. 0.00350
5. 4.2435

ANSWERS TO PROBLEMS ON PAGE 3
DIVIDING DECIMALS (D)

1. 1.3533
2. 20
3. 26
4. 145.4545 = 145.455
5. 30

ANSWERS TO PROBLEMS ON PAGE 3
PROPORTIONS

1. 24
2. 3.25
3. 9.6
4. 0.25

1

REVIEW OF ARITHMETIC

Calculations of drugs and solutions require a basic understanding of whole numbers, fractions, and decimals. It is helpful to review this material. This section covers the basic rules for working with fractions, decimals, and percentages. It can be used as a review for those areas in which you were weak in the pretest.

1. A fraction is a part of a whole number. It consists of a numerator, which is the top number, and a denominator, which is the bottom number.

   In the fraction $\frac{3}{4}$, 3 is the _____,

   numerator

   and 4 is the _____.

   denominator

2. Fractions should always be reduced to the lowest term. To do this, the numerator and the denominator are each divided by the largest number by which they are both divisible.

   In the fraction $\frac{8}{24}$, both the numerator and denominator are divisible by eight,

   so $\frac{8}{24}$ = _____.

   $\frac{1}{3}$

3. To change a mixed number (a whole number and a fraction) to a fraction, the whole number is multiplied by the denominator of the fraction. This number is added to the numerator of the fraction and the sum is placed over the denominator.

$2\frac{1}{6}$ = (2 × _____) + 1

So $2\frac{1}{6}$ = $\dfrac{\rule{3cm}{0.4pt}}{6}$.

6

13

4. To change an improper fraction (a fraction whose numerator is greater than its denominator, and therefore, whose value is greater than 1) to a mixed number, the numerator is divided by the denominator. Anything that is not further divisible is expressed as a fraction.

$\dfrac{13}{6}$ = 6$\overline{)13}$ = _____

$2\frac{1}{6}$

5. To add fractions with the same denominator, add the numerators and place that sum over the denominator. The answer is reduced to the lowest term if necessary.

$\dfrac{4}{7} + \dfrac{2}{7}$ = _____

$\dfrac{6}{7}$

6. To add fractions with different denominators, first find the lowest number evenly divisible by both. This is called the "lowest common denominator." Convert each fraction to the same terms by dividing the denominator into the lowest common denominator and multiplying that answer and the numerator. The answer to this is the new numerator. The numerators are then added together and placed over the lowest common denominator.

In the problem $\frac{1}{6} + \frac{3}{4}$, the lowest common denominator of $\frac{1}{6}$ and $\frac{3}{4}$ is

_____.

Therefore, $\frac{1}{6} = \dfrac{}{12}$ and $\frac{3}{4} = \dfrac{}{12}$.

So $\frac{1}{6} + \frac{3}{4} = $ _____.

(The fraction should be reduced to the lowest term.)

12

2

9

$\frac{11}{12}$

---

7. To subtract fractions with the same denominator, subtract the numerators and place the answer over the denominator. The answer should be reduced to the lowest term.

$\frac{3}{4} - \frac{1}{4} = $ _____

$\frac{2}{4} = \frac{1}{2}$

8. To subtract fractions with different denominators, the lowest common denominator must first be found and the fractions must be converted as in frame 6. The numerators are then subtracted and placed over the lowest common denominator and reduced to the lowest term.

In the problem $\frac{5}{7} - \frac{1}{3}$, the lowest common denominator of $\frac{5}{7}$ and $\frac{1}{3}$ is _____.

$\frac{5}{7} = \dfrac{\rule{1cm}{0.4pt}}{21}$.

$\frac{1}{3} = \dfrac{\rule{1cm}{0.4pt}}{21}$.

So $\frac{5}{7} - \frac{1}{3} =$ _____.

21

15

7

$\frac{8}{21}$

---

9. To multiply fractions, multiply the numerators together. The answer is the new numerator. Then multiply the denominators; that number is the new denominator.

In the problem $\frac{7}{8} \times \frac{1}{2}$,

$7 \times 1 =$ _____

$8 \times 2 =$ _____.

So $\frac{7}{8} \times \frac{1}{2} =$ _____.

7

16

$\frac{7}{16}$

---

10. To divide fractions, the division problem must be changed to a multiplication problem. Do this by inverting the divisor (the number to the right of the division sign) and then following the rule for multiplication. The answer should be reduced to the lowest term.

In the problem $\frac{1}{8} \div 3$, the 3, the 3 is changed to _____, and the two fractions are multiplied.

$\frac{1}{8} \times \frac{1}{3} =$ _____

$\frac{1}{3}$

$\frac{1}{24}$

11. A decimal represents a fraction whose denominator is a multiple of 10.

.10 is the same as the fraction $\frac{1}{10}$.

.01 is the same as the fraction

_____.

$\frac{1}{100}$

---

12. When multiplying decimals, the two numbers are treated as whole numbers. The answer must have as many numbers to the right of the decimal point as the *total* number of decimal points in the numbers being multiplied.

3.4 × 1.31 will have _____ numbers to the right of the decimal point.

3

3.4 × 1.31 = _____

4.454

---

13. To divide two decimals, the decimal point of the divisor is moved to the right until the number is a whole number. The decimal point of the dividend (the number to the left of the division sign) must be moved an equal number of places.

3 ÷ .02 = .02⟌3.00

2⟌300 = _____

150

---

14. The term percent (%) means parts per hundred. To change a percent to a decimal, the % symbol is dropped and the number is divided by 100.

20% is the same as the decimal

_____.

.20

15. When calculating with percentages, the % sign is dropped, the number is changed to a decimal, and rules pertaining to decimals are followed.

16. A ratio expresses the comparison of one number with another.

A ratio expressing the relationship of three to four is written with a colon between the two numbers ($3:4$) or as a fraction ($\frac{3}{4}$).

The ratio expressing the relationship of

7 to 8 can be written _____ or

_____.

$7:8$

$\frac{7}{8}$

17. A proportion is a statement of two ratios that are equal. An example is

$\frac{1}{5} = \frac{20}{100}$. It is read, _____ is

equal to 20 to 100.

1 to 5

18. One number in a proportion may be missing. The missing number is replaced by an x.

For example, $\frac{2}{3} = \frac{x}{12}$. It is necessary to find the value of x.

To find the value of x, cross multiply.

$\frac{2}{3} = \frac{x}{12}$

$2 \times 12 = 3x$

_____ $= 3x$

24

$x = 24 \div 3$

$x =$ _____

8

12

19. Solve for x in the following problem.

$$\frac{3}{7} = \frac{12}{x}$$

$3x = 7 \times 12$

$3x = $ _____   84

$x = $ _____   28

Following are some practice problems.

PRACTICE PROBLEMS

REVIEW OF ARITHMETIC

(ANSWERS ON PAGE 14)

1. $\frac{5}{6} + \frac{6}{6} =$

2. $\frac{3}{14} + \frac{13}{14} =$

3. $3\frac{1}{4} + \frac{5}{6} =$

4. $2\frac{5}{16} + 4\frac{1}{5} =$

5. $2\frac{2}{5} - \frac{3}{4} =$

6. $\frac{14}{15} - \frac{2}{3} =$

7. $\frac{1}{12} \times \frac{3}{5} =$

8. $\frac{8}{9} \times \frac{3}{4} =$

9. $\frac{9}{10} \div 4 =$

10. $\frac{7}{8} \div \frac{2}{3} =$

11. $3.25 \times 7.03 =$

12. $9.12 \times 1.25 =$

13. $12 \div 3.2 =$

14. $4.25 \div 3.1 =$

15. $13 \times 20\% =$

16. $6.2 \times 31\% =$

17. $24 \div 8\% =$

18. $\frac{1}{6} = \frac{x}{24}$

19. $\frac{4}{9} = \frac{8}{x}$

20. $\frac{3}{5} = \frac{x}{25}$

ANSWERS TO PROBLEMS ON PAGE 13

REVIEW OF ARITHMETIC

1. $\dfrac{11}{6} = 1\dfrac{5}{6}$

2. $\dfrac{16}{14} = 1\dfrac{2}{14} = 1\dfrac{1}{7}$

3. $\dfrac{39}{12} + \dfrac{10}{12} = \dfrac{49}{12} = 4\dfrac{1}{12}$

4. $\dfrac{185}{80} + \dfrac{336}{80} = \dfrac{521}{80} = 6\dfrac{41}{80}$

5. $\dfrac{48}{20} - \dfrac{15}{20} = \dfrac{33}{20} = 1\dfrac{13}{20}$

6. $\dfrac{14}{15} - \dfrac{10}{15} = \dfrac{4}{15}$

7. $\dfrac{3}{60} = \dfrac{1}{20}$

8. $\dfrac{24}{36} = \dfrac{2}{3}$

9. $\dfrac{9}{10} \times \dfrac{1}{4} = \dfrac{9}{40}$

10. $\dfrac{7}{8} \times \dfrac{3}{2} = \dfrac{21}{16} = 1\dfrac{5}{16}$

11. 22.8475

12. 11.4000

13. $32\overline{)120} = 3.75$

14. $31\overline{)42.5} = 1.371$

15. $13 \times .20 = 2.60$

16. $6.2 \times .31 = 1.922$

17. $8\overline{)2400} = 300$

18. $x = 4$

19. $x = 18$

20. $x = 15$

2

THE METRIC SYSTEM

The first step in learning about the mathematics of drugs and solutions is to become familiar with the various systems and units used in measuring drugs and solutions. The first of these systems is the *metric* system of weights and measures. This system was developed in France in the latter part of the eighteenth century and is the one used in most European countries. Today, the metric system is utilized in hospitals throughout the United States. In the metric system, fractional quantities (i.e., less than one) are expressed as decimals. For example, one-half is written as 0.5. In this system, the unit of length is the meter (hence "metric").

The units which a nurse will use in measuring medication are (1) by weight—the kilogram, the gram, and the milligram; and (2) by volume—the liter and the milliliter or the cubic centimeter. (Although the milliliter and the cubic centimeter are not exactly equal, the difference is so slight that the terms are used interchangeably.)

This chapter will examine the relationships between these units for weight and volume and will show how quantities are expressed within the framework of the metric system.

---

1. When administering medications to the patient, the nurse will use one of three systems of measurement. The first of these that we will discuss is the international decimal system called the <u>metric system</u>.

The _____ _____ is the international decimal system of weights and measures.

metric system

---

2. In the metric system, fractions are expressed as decimals. In the decimal system, the fraction one-half is written as 0.5.

Four-tenths is written as _____.

0.4

---

3. The unit of weight in the metric system is expressed in terms of the gram (g).

The _____ is said to be the unit of weight in the metric system.

gram

---

4. In the metric system, five grams is written 5.0 grams or 5.0 g.

Ten grams is written as 10.0 g or

_____ _____.

10.0 grams

---

5. The prefix "kilo" indicates 1,000.0. A

kilogram (kg) is _____ grams.

1,000.0

---

6. To change kilograms to grams, multiply the number of kilograms by 1,000 or move the decimal three places to the right.
Thus:
5.0 kilograms (kg) × 1,000 =
    5,000.0 grams (g) or
5.0 kilograms (kg) = 5.000 =
    5,000.0 grams (g)

10.0 kg = _____ g

10,000.0

---

7. 400.0 kg = 400,000.0 g

25.0 kg = _____ g

25,000.0

---

8. 2.0 kg = _____ g

2,000.0

9. To change grams to kilograms, <u>divide</u> the number of grams by 1,000 or move the decimal three places to the <u>left</u>. Thus:

1,000.0 g ÷ 1,000 = 1.0 kg or

1,000.0 g = 1 000.0 = 1.0 kg

4,000.0 g = _____ kg

4.0

---

10. 60.0 g = 0.06 kg

75.0 g = _____ kg

0.075

---

11. 750.0 g = _____ kg

0.75

---

12. The prefix <u>milli</u> indicates one one-thousandth of the unit. A milligram (mg) is

_____ g.

one one-thousandth

---

13. One one-thousandth gram may also be

written _____ g.

0.001

---

14. 4.0 mg = 0.004 g

13.0 mg = _____ g

0.013

---

15. 230.0 mg = _____ g

0.23

---

16. To change grams to milligrams, <u>multiply</u> the number of grams by 1,000 or move the decimal three places to the <u>right</u>.

3.0 g × 1,000 = 3,000.0 mg or

3.0 g = 3.000 = 3,000.0 mg

2.0 g = _____ mg

2,000.0

---

17. 15.0 g = 15,000.0 mg

35.0 g = _____ mg

35,000.0

---

18. 1.5 g = _____ mg

1,500.0

19. To change milligrams to grams, <u>divide</u> the number of milligrams by <u>1,000</u> or move the decimal three places to the <u>left</u>.
Thus:
1,200.0 mg ÷ 1,000 = 1.2 g or
1,200.0 mg = 1 200.0 = 1.2 g

50.0 mg = _____ g

0.05

---

20. 14.0 mg = 0.014 g

100.0 mg = _____ g

0.10

---

21. 250.0 mg = _____ g

0.25

---

22. Volume in the metric system is expressed in terms of the <u>liter</u>. The

_____ is the unit of volume in the metric system.

liter

---

23. The nurse will most frequently use the <u>liter</u> and the <u>milliliter</u> (ml). You will recall that the prefix <u>milli</u> means one one-thousandth of a unit. Here the prefix <u>milli</u>

indicates _____ _____ of a liter.

one one-thousandth

---

24. One <u>milliliter</u> (ml) and one <u>cubic centimeter</u> (cc) are considered equivalent.

Therefore, 10.0 ml and _____ cc can be used interchangeably.

10.0

---

25. To change liters to milliliters (ml) <u>multiply</u> the number of liters by <u>1,000</u> or move the decimal three places to the <u>right</u>.
Thus:
2.0 liters × 1,000 = 2,000.0 ml (or cc)
or
2.0 liters = 2.000 = 2,000.0 ml (or cc)

10.0 liters = _____ ml (or cc)

10,000.0

26. 15.0 liters = 15,000.0 ml (or cc)

33.0 liters = _____ ml (or cc) | 33,000.0

27. 4.0 liters = _____ ml (or cc) | 4,000.0

28. To change milliliters (or cubic centimeters) to liters, <u>divide</u> the number of milliliters by 1,000 or move the decimal three places to the <u>left</u>.
Thus:
1,500.0 ml ÷ 1,000 = 1.5 liters or
1,500.0 ml = 1 500.0 = 1.5 liters

15.0 cc = _____ liters | 0.015

29. 18.0 cc = 0.018 liters

250.0 cc = _____ liters | 0.25

30. 965.0 cc = _____ liters | 0.965

Here are a few problems to review what you have just learned.

PRACTICE PROBLEMS
METRIC SYSTEM
(ANSWERS ON PAGE 20)

1. 0.25 liters = _____ ml

2. 4.0 liters = _____ ml

3. 500.0 ml = _____ liters

4. 1,320.0 ml = _____ liters

5. 8.0 mg = _____ g

6. 750.0 mg = __.75__ g

7. 10.0 g = _____ mg

8. 3.0 g = _____ mg

9. 154.0 cc = _____ liters

10. 1.75 liters = _____ cc

ANSWERS TO PROBLEMS ON PAGE 19
METRIC SYSTEM

1. 250.0

2. 4,000.0

3. 0.5

4. 1.32

5. 0.008

6. 0.75

7. 10,000.0

8. 3,000.0

9. 0.154

10. 1,750.0

3

THE APOTHECARIES' SYSTEM

The apothecaries' system is the system of weights and measures which was traditionally used in the United States to dispense drugs. This system dates back to early colonial days and was part of the system of weights and measures then in use in England. At that time, the unit "grain" was considered the weight of a grain of wheat, and the "minim" was the quantity of water equal to the weight of a grain of wheat. Today, the apothecaries' system is not used as frequently as the metric system.

Units of weight used to measure drugs in the apothecaries' system are the grain, the dram, and the ounce. Fluid volume is measured by the minim, the fluidram, the fluidounce, the pint, and the quart. The terms fluidram and fluidounce are usually shortened to dram and ounce with the understanding that drugs in liquid form would be measured by volume and those in solid form would be measured by weight.

As you work through this chapter you will learn the proper notation for this system and the relationships between the various units.

---

1. The second system we will consider is the apothecaries' system. This was the original system used in the United States. In medicine today the apothecaries' system is largely being replaced by the metric system. However, it is important for the nurse to understand both the metric and the

   _____ systems.

   apothecaries'

---

2. In the apothecaries' system, quantities less than one are expressed as common fractions. One-tenth is written $\frac{1}{10}$. Therefore, three-fourths is written _____.

$\frac{3}{4}$

---

3. An exception to this rule is the frequent writing of one-half as ss (Latin "semis"). In the apothecaries' system, one-half is written _____.

ss

---

4. <u>Notations</u> in the apothecaries' system use lower-case Roman numerals: i (1), v (5), x (10), l (50), c (100). Five and one-half is written vss.

One and one-half is written _____.

iss

---

5. Seven and one-half is written _____.

viiss

---

6. Arabic numbers are used in <u>working problems</u> in the apothecaries' system, rather than lower case Roman numerals.

When working problems in the apothecaries' system, _____ numerals are used.

Arabic

---

7. Mixed numbers other than those containing one-half are written with the number and the fraction. Three and three-fourths is written as $3\frac{3}{4}$. Therefore, two and one-fourth would be written _____.

$2\frac{1}{4}$

8. The most commonly used unit for weight of medications in the apothecaries' system is the <u>grain</u> (gr). The unit of measure is placed before the numeral: five grains is written grains v or gr v.

Ten grains is written _____ or

_____ .

grains x

gr x

---

9. Six and one-half grains is written

_____ or _____ .

grains viss; gr viss

---

10. $\frac{1}{200}$ of a grain is written _____ .

grains $\frac{1}{200}$ or gr $\frac{1}{200}$

---

11. Volume in the apothecaries' system is expressed as minims (M.), drams (ʒ), ounce (℥), pint (pt.), and quart (qt.).

If minims (M.) lx (60) = drams (ʒ) i, then minims (M.) cxx (120) = drams

(ʒ) _____ .

ii

---

12. If drams (ʒ) iii = minims (M.) clxxx,

then drams (ʒ) iv = minims (M.)

_____ .

ccxl (240)

---

13. In the following conversions, use Arabic numbers.

ʒ2 = M. _____

120

---

14. ʒ8 = ounce (℥) 1,

therefore, ʒ32 = ℥_____ .

4

---

15. If ʒ40 = ℥5,

then ʒ20 = ℥_____ .

$2\frac{1}{2}$

---

16. If ℥2 = ℥16,

then ℥3 = ℥_____.

24

17. ℥6 = ℥_____.

48

18. There are 16 ounces in one pint (pt.).

If ℥16 = pt.1

then ℥8 = pt. _____.

$\dfrac{1}{2}$

19. ℥32 = pt. _____

2

20. If pt. 3 = ℥48,

then pt. 5 = ℥_____.

80

21. pt. 10 = ℥_____

160

22. There are two pints in one quart (qt.).

If pt. 2 = qt. 1

then pt. 4 = qt. _____.

2

23. pt. 3 = qt. _____.

$1\dfrac{1}{2}$

24. If qt. 6 = pt. 12

then qt. 12 = pt. _____.

24

25. qt. $2\dfrac{1}{2}$ = pt. _____

5

On the next page are a few problems to review what you have just learned.

PRACTICE PROBLEMS

APOTHECARIES' SYSTEM

(ANSWERS ON PAGE 26)

---

1. ℥ivss = ℨ_____

2. ℨviii = ℥_____

3. M. lx = ℨ_____

4. ℨxii = ℥_____

5. pt. ss = ℥_____

6. qt. 2 = pt. _____

7. M xxx = ℨ_____

8. pt. vi = qt. _____

9. ℥viii = ℨ_____

10. ℨiv = M. _____

APOTHECARIES' SYSTEM

---

1. 36

2. 1

3. 1

4. $1\frac{1}{2}$

5. 8

6. 4

7. ss $\left(\frac{1}{2}\right)$

8. 3

9. 64

10. 240

4

HOUSEHOLD MEASUREMENTS

Household measurements are those commonly used in everyday home situations. You will recognize these measurements as those you have used in following recipes and in shopping in the supermarket. Household measurements are not as accurate as those of the metric and the apothecaries' systems and, therefore, are not used to pour medications when either of the other systems is available. If you examine spoons, cups, and glasses in your own home, it will be evident to you that there is considerable variation in capacity. You, as a nurse, may find that the household measurement may be the only one you have to go by when working in a home situation or that it is the easiest system to use in patient teaching. These are measurements with which the patient is familiar, and there are situations in which they may be used with safety, such as "normal saline solution" for a gargle.

---

1. Household <u>measurements</u> are not as accurate as metric or apothecaries' system measurements and therefore are not used as frequently in medicine. However, the home-care nurse often will find accurate measures not available and must use what is available.

   Household measures are not as desirable as metric or apothecaries' measures because they are less

   _____.

   accurate

2. Sixty <u>drops</u> (gtt) are considered <u>one</u> <u>teaspoonful</u> (t.).

60 gtt (drops) = 1 t. (teaspoonful)

Therefore, 120 gtt = _____ t.

2

---

3. 5 t. = 300 gtt

3 t. = _____ gtt

180

---

4. 30 gtt = _____ t.

$\frac{1}{2}$

---

5. Three <u>teaspoonfuls</u> (t.) equal <u>one</u> <u>table-spoonful</u> (T.).

3 t. (teaspoonfuls) = 1 T. (tablespoon-ful)

9 t. = _____ T.

3

---

6. 6 T. = 18 t.

4 T. = _____ t.

12

---

7. 6 t. = _____ T.

2

---

8. Two <u>tablespoonfuls</u> (T.) equal <u>one</u> <u>fluid</u> <u>ounce</u>.

2 T. = 1 ounce (the word fluid is usually omitted)

4 T. = _____ ounces.

2

---

9. 5 ounces = 10 T.

4 ounces = _____ T.

8

---

10. 12 T. = _____ ounces.

6

---

11. Eight <u>fluid</u> <u>ounces</u> equal <u>one</u> <u>cupful</u>.

8 ounces = 1 cupful

16 ounces = _____ cupfuls.

2

12. 10 cupfuls = 80 ounces.	
3 cupfuls = _____ ounces.	24
13. 48 ounces = _____ cupfuls.	6
14. <u>Two</u> <u>pints</u> (pt.) equal <u>one</u> <u>quart</u> (qt.). 2 pt. (pints) = 1 qt. (quart) Therefore, 4 pt. = _____ qt.	2
15. 5 qt. = 10 pt. 3 qt. = _____ pt.	6
16. 10 qt. = _____ pt.	20

PRACTICE PROBLEMS

HOUSEHOLD MEASUREMENTS

(ANSWERS ON PAGE 30)

1. 3 T. = _____ ounces

2. 5 ounces = _____ T.

3. 6 cupfuls = _____ ounces

4. 4 quarts = _____ pints

5. 6 t. = _____ T.

6. 12 ounces = _____ cupfuls

7. 3 cupfuls = _____ ounces

8. 3 T. = _____ t.

9. 4 t. = _____ gtt

HOUSEHOLD MEASUREMENTS

---

1. $1\frac{1}{2}$

2. 10

3. 48

4. 8

5. 2

6. $1\frac{1}{2}$

7. 24

8. 9

9. 240

5

EQUIVALENTS

By definition, an equivalent is a given quantity which is considered to be of equal value to a quantity that is expressed in a different system. In comparing the metric, the apothecaries', and the household systems, you will find that a unit of one system never exactly equals a unit of another system. For example, while 1 ounce is exactly 29.5729 grams, in working dosage problems, you will round off to the nearest whole number. Hence, 30 grams is the approximate equivalent of 1 ounce.

By using the approximate equivalent in computation, you will obtain a slightly different answer than if you used the exact equivalent; however, a difference of 10 percent or less is considered legitimate.

Because these three systems of weights and measures are currently in use in the United States, it is most important that you not only thoroughly understand each of the systems, but that you be able to convert from one to another accurately and without hesitation.

1. There will be times when the three measurement systems will have to be used interchangeably. The order for the drug may be in metric terms, and the method of measurement available in _____ or _____ systems.	apothecaries' household
2. An equivalent is an amount in one system which may be substituted for a like amount in another system. However, the _____ may not be exactly equal to the original measure.	equivalent

3. For example, 1.0 g is exactly equal to 15.432 grains. In computing dosages of medications, however, the nurse will substitute 15 grains for 1.0 grams when necessary.

We can say that grains 15 is the

_____ of 1.0 grams.   equivalent

---

4. When it is necessary to convert from one system to another, it doesn't matter if the desired dose or the on-hand dose is the one which is converted. Most nurses find it simpler to convert the desired dose to that on hand; therefore, in this text we will convert

the _____ _____ to the   desired dose

dose on hand.

---

5. To change <u>grams</u> to <u>grains</u>, multiply the number of grams by 15.

grams × 15 = _____   grains

---

6. Example:
How many grains are in 2.0 grams?

grams × 15 = grains

2.0 grams × 15 = grains _____   30

---

7. Example:
0.5 g is how many grains?

0.5 g × 15 = gr _____ $7\frac{1}{2}$

---

8. 30 grams is how many grains?

30.0 g = gr _____   450

---

9. 3.0 grams is how many grains?

3.0 g = gr _____   45

10. 0.05 grams is how many grains?

0.05 g = gr _____

0.75

---

11. To change <u>grains</u> to <u>grams</u>, divide the number of grains by 15.

grains ÷ 15 = _____

grams

---

12. Example:
45 grains is how many grams?

grains ÷ 15 = grams

gr 45 ÷ 15 = _____ grams

3.0

---

13. Example:
grains 5 is what part of a gram?

gr 5 ÷ 15 = _____ grams

0.3

---

14. grains iii is how many grams?

gr iii = _____ g

0.2

---

15. grain $\frac{1}{4}$ is how many grams?

gr $\frac{1}{4}$ = _____ g

0.016

---

16. In computing dosages of medications, 30.0 grams is considered the equivalent of ℥i.

Therefore, we can say _____ g is ℥i.

30.0

---

17. To change <u>grams</u> to <u>ounces</u>, divide the number of grams by 30.

grams ÷ 30 = _____

ounces

18. Example:

In 60.0 grams there are how many ounces?

grams ÷ 30 = ounces

60.0 g ÷ 30 = ounces _____   2

---

19. Example:

How many ounces are in 150.0 grams?

150.0 g ÷ 30 = ounces _____   5

---

20. How many ounces are in 30 grams?

30 g ÷ 30 = ounces _____   1

---

21. How many ounces are in 135 grams?

135 g ÷ 30 = ounces _____ $4\frac{1}{2}$

---

22. To change <u>ounces</u> to <u>grams</u>, multiply the number of ounces by 30.

ounces × 30 = _____   grams

---

23. Example:

How many grams are in 4 ounces?

ounces × 30 = grams

ʒ4 × 30 = _____   120.0

---

24. Example:

How many grams are in ounces viss?

$ʒ6\frac{1}{2}$ × 30 = _____   195.0

---

25. How many grams are in ounces iii?

ʒ3 × 30 = _____   90.0

---

26. How many grams are in ounces xx?

ʒ20 × 30 = _____   600.0

27. 30.0 cc is considered the equivalent of ℥i. In converting from metric to apothecaries' systems the nurse will consider

_____ cc as being equal to ℥i.

30.0

---

28. To change <u>cc</u> to <u>ounces</u>, divide the number of cc by 30.

cc ÷ 30 = _____

ounces

---

29. Example:

240.0 cc is how many ounces?

cc ÷ 30 = ounces

240.0 cc ÷ 30 = ℥_____

8

---

30. Example:

How many ounces are there in 180.0 cc?

180.0 cc ÷ 30 = ℥_____

6

---

31. How many ounces are in 60.0 cc?

60.0 cc ÷ 30 = ℥_____

2

---

32. How many ounces are in 1,000.0 cc?

1,000.0 cc ÷ 30 = ℥_____

$33\frac{1}{3}$

---

33. To change <u>ounces</u> to <u>cc</u> multiply the number of ounces by 30.

ounces × 30 = _____

cc

---

34. Example:

A four-ounce bottle holds how many cc?

ounces × 30 = cc

℥4 × 30 = _____ cc

120.0

35. Example:
How many cc are in 10 ounces?

$10 \times 30 =$ _____ cc

300.0

---

36. How many cc are in 6 ounces?

$6 \times 30 =$ _____ cc

180.0

---

37. How many cc are in $2\frac{1}{2}$ ounces?

$2\frac{1}{2} =$ _____ cc

. 75.0

---

38. In working problems, 1.0 cc is equivalent to minims xv. Therefore, 1.0 cc may

be substituted for M. _____.

15

---

39. To change <u>cc</u> to <u>minims</u>, multiply the number of cc by 15.

cc $\times$ 15 = _____

minims

---

40. Example:
In 15.0 cc there are how many minims?

cc $\times$ 15 = minims

5.0 cc $\times$ 15 = M. _____

225

---

41. Example:
How many minims are in 5 cubic centimeters?

5.0 cc $\times$ 15 = M. _____

75

---

42. Example:
Using the equivalent 1.0 cc = 15 M., solve the following:

In 2.0 cc there are _____ M.

30

---

43. Example:
In 3.5 cc there are _____ M.

$52\frac{1}{2}$

44. In 3.0 cc there are _____ M.	45
45. In 7.0 cc there are _____ M.	105
46. To change <u>minims</u> to <u>cc</u>, divide the number of minims by 15. minims ÷ 15 = _____	cc
47. Example: How many cc are there in 45 minims? minims ÷ 15 = cc M. 45 ÷ 15 = _____ cc	3.0
48. Example: How would you measure 60 minims in a medicine glass marked only in cc? M. 60 ÷ 15 = _____ cc	4.0
49. How many cc are there in 30 minims? M. 30 ÷ 15 = _____ cc	2.0
50. How many cc are there in lxviiss minims? M. $67\frac{1}{2}$ ÷ 15 = _____ cc	4.5
51. The metric equivalent of gr i is 60.0 mg. In working problems, the nurse will substitute _____ mg for gr i.	60.0
52. To change <u>milligrams</u> to <u>grains</u>, divide the number of milligrams by 60. milligrams ÷ 60 = _____	grains

53. Example:

How many grains are in 600.0 mg?

milligrams ÷ 60 = grains

600.0 mg ÷ 60 = gr _____   10

---

54. Example:

How many grains are in 20.0 mg?

20.0 mg ÷ 60 = gr _____ $\frac{1}{3}$

---

55. Example:

10.0 mg is how many grains?

10.0 mg ÷ 60 = gr _____ $\frac{1}{6}$

---

56. 0.3 mg is how many grains?

0.3 mg ÷ 60 = gr _____   gr $\frac{1}{200}$

---

57. To change <u>grains</u> to <u>milligrams</u>, multiply the number of grains by 60.

grains × 60 = _____   milligrams

---

58. Example:

How many milligrams are in gr xii?

grains × 60 = milligrams

gr 12 × 60 = _____ mg   720

---

59. Example:

How many milligrams are in gr ss?

gr $\frac{1}{2}$ × 60 = _____ mg   30

---

60. Example:

Gr ii is how many milligrams?

gr 2 × 60 = _____ mg   120

---

61. Gr $\frac{1}{200}$ is how many milligrams?

gr $\frac{1}{200}$ × 60 = _____ mg   0.3

---

62. Gr ix is how many milligrams?

gr 9 × 60 = _____ mg

| 540

63. In computing dosages for some medications, weight in kilograms is used. A kilogram is equivalent to 2.2 pounds. Therefore, we can say 2.2 pounds is

equivalent to _____ kilogram (kg).

| 1

64. To change pounds to kilograms, divide the number of pounds by 2.2

pounds ÷ 2.2 = _____

| kilograms

65. Example:
How many kilograms are in 220 pounds?

pounds ÷ 2.2 = kg

220 pounds ÷ 2.2 = _____ kg

| 100.0

66. Example:
How many kilograms are in 15 pounds?

15 pounds ÷ 2.2 = _____ kg

| 6.8

67. How many kilograms are in 44 pounds?

44 pounds ÷ 2.2 = _____ kg

| 20

68. How many kilograms are in 198 pounds?

198 pounds ÷ 2.2 = _____ kg

| 90

69. To change kilograms to pounds, multiply the number of kilograms by 2.2.

kilograms × 2.2 = _____

| pounds

70. Example:
How many pounds are equivalent to 60 kilograms?

kilograms × 2.2 = pounds

60 kg × 2.2 = _____ pounds   132

---

71. Example:
How many pounds are equivalent to 20 kilograms?

20 kg × 2.2 = _____ pounds   44

---

72. How many pounds are equivalent to 500 kilograms?

500 kg × 2.2 = _____ pounds   1100

---

73. How many pounds are equivalent to 9 kilograms?

9 kg × 2.2 = _____ pounds   19.8

---

74. The metric equivalent of 1 inch is 2.54 cm. To change inches to cm, multiply

by _____.   2.54

---

75. To change cm to inches, the nurse

must _____ by 2.54.   divide

---

76. How many cm is $3\frac{1}{2}$ inches?

$3\frac{1}{2}$ × 2.54 = _____   8.89 cm

---

77. How many cm is $\frac{1}{2}$ inch?

$\frac{1}{2}$ × 2.54 = _____   1.27 cm

---

78. How many inches is 3 cm?

3 ÷ 2.54 = _____   1.18 inches

79. How many inches is 12 cm?

12 ÷ 2.54 = _____

4.72 inches

---

80. It may be necessary to change a temperature from Celsius (°C) scale to Fahrenheit (°F) scale. To convert a Celsius (°C) reading to Fahrenheit (°F), use the formula:

$°F = \dfrac{9}{5} °C + 32°$.

If the °C reading is 37°, the °F is

$\dfrac{9}{5} (37°) + 32° =$ _____.

98.6°F

---

81. A Celsius temperature of 50° is

_____ °F.

122

---

82. To change a temperature from Fahrenheit (°F) to Celsius (°C), use the formula:

$°C = \dfrac{5}{9}(°F - 32°)$.

If the temperature is 100°F, the °C temperature is

$\dfrac{5}{9}(100° - 32°) =$ _____.

38°C

---

83. A temperature of 160°F would be

_____ °C.

71.1

On page 43 are problems to review what you have just learned.

PRACTICE PROBLEMS

EQUIVALENTS

(ANSWERS ON PAGE 44)

---

1. 15.0 g = gr ___325___

2. 15.0 cc = ℥_____

3. 40.0 g = ℥_____ .

4. M. xl = _____ cc

5. 80.0 mg = gr _____

6. ℥xii = _____ g

7. gr iv = ___240___ mg

8. gr xi = ___15___ g

9. ℥viiss = _____ cc

10. 20.0 cc = M. _____

11. 35 pounds = _____ kg

12. 78 kg = _____ pounds

13. 3.2 g = gr ___48.___

14. gr v = _____ g

15. 70 g = ℥_____

16. ℥lxi = _____ g

17. 105 cc = ℥_____

18. ℥xxx = _____ cc

19. 10 cc = M. _____

20. M. xc = _____ cc

21. 300 mg = gr _____

22. gr $\frac{1}{4}$ = ___15___ mg

23. 132 pounds = _____ kg

24. 72 kg = _____ pounds

25. 94°F = _____ °C

26. 72°C = _____ °F

27. 57°C = _____ °F

28. 20°F = _____ °C

29. 3.25 inches = _____ cm

30. 16 inches = _____ cm

31. 21 cm = _____ inches

32. 1 cm = _____ inches

ANSWERS TO PROBLEMS ON PAGE 43

EQUIVALENTS

1. 225
2. $\frac{1}{2}$
3. $1\frac{1}{3}$
4. 2.67
5. $1\frac{1}{3}$
6. 360.0
7. 240.0
8. 0.73
9. 225.0
10. 300
11. 15.9 or 16
12. 171.6 or 172
13. 48
14. 0.3
15. $2\frac{1}{3}$
16. 1,830

17. $3\frac{1}{2}$
18. 900
19. 150
20. 6.0
21. 5
22. 15.0
23. 60
24. 158.4
25. 34.4
26. 161.6
27. 134.6
28. −6.7
29. 8.26
30. 40.64
31. 8.27
32. 0.39

6

ORAL MEDICATIONS

The most common method of administering medications is by mouth. This is considered the safest method and is usually the easiest for both the client and the nurse. Medications to be given p.o. (Latin per os—by mouth) come in varied forms: pills, tablets, capsules, powders, and liquids.

The dose of medication that is available is frequently different from the dose to be given. Therefore, it will be necessary to calculate how many or what part of this oral medication must be given in order to administer the correct dose. Many tablets are scored so that they may be easily broken into halves or quarters. Medications that are soluble in water may be dissolved to divide the dose.

1. In preparing to administer oral medications, the nurse may find that the prescribed dose is different from what is available. When the size of the prescribed _____ and that of the medication on hand are not the same, the nurse must determine how much of the available medication must be given.	dose
2. If the size of the tablet on hand is larger than the prescribed dose, less than one _____ will be needed.	tablet

3. If the size of the tablet on hand is smaller than the prescribed dose, _____ than one tablet will be used.

more

4. To calculate the part of a tablet to be used or the _____ _____, the nurse will use the formula given in frame 5.

number of tablets

5. Formula:

$$\frac{\text{Desired dose}}{\text{On-hand dose}} \text{ or } \frac{D}{H}$$

The desired dose (D) is the _____ of medication prescribed.

amount or quantity

6. To solve the formula $\frac{D}{H}$

the quantity D is _____ by the quantity H.

divided

7. Example:
The order is for 500 mg of chlorpropamide.
On hand is:
chlorpropamide (Diabinese) 250 mg.
How much of the tablet(s) would you use?

Use the formula $\frac{D}{H}$ and substitute known values: $\dfrac{\underline{?}\ \text{mg}}{\underline{?}\ \text{mg}}$

500
250

8. $\dfrac{D}{H} = \dfrac{500\ \text{mg}}{250\ \text{mg}} = 500\ \text{mg} \div 250\ \text{mg} =$

_____ of the 250-mg tablets will be used.

2

9. Another way to solve the formula $\frac{D}{H}$ is to reduce the fraction to its lowest terms:

$$\frac{D}{H} = \frac{500 \text{ mg}}{250 \text{ mg}} = \underline{\quad \frac{?}{?} \quad}$$

2 mg
1 mg

---

10. $\frac{2}{1} = $ _____ of the 250-mg tablets will be used.

2

---

11. The nurse should use the method that she finds easiest, or she may use the two _____ interchangeably.

methods

---

12. Example:
The order is for furosemide 20 mg.
On hand is:
furosemide (Lasix) 40 mg tablet.

$$\frac{D}{H} = \frac{\underline{?} \text{ mg}}{\underline{?} \text{ mg}}$$

Substitute the known values.

20
40

---

13. $\frac{D}{H} = \frac{20 \text{ mg}}{40 \text{ mg}} = \frac{1}{2}$

or _____ tablet of furosemide 40 mg will be used.

$\frac{1}{2}$

---

14. Using the alternative method:

$$\frac{D}{H} = \frac{20 \text{ mg}}{40 \text{ mg}} = 20 \text{ mg} \div 40 \text{ mg} =$$

_____ tablet(s) of furosemide 40 mg will be used.

$\frac{1}{2}$

15. When oral liquids are ordered, use the formula:

$$\frac{\text{Desired dose}}{\text{On-hand dose}} \times \text{Volume or } \frac{D}{H} \times V.$$

The container will be labeled according to the amount of the drug in a given volume of the liquid. In this case the amount of drug in a given volume will be the _____ of the formula $\frac{D}{H} \times V.$

D

---

16. Example:
The label indicates that there are 125 mg of cloxacillin per 5 cc. How will you give 250 mg?

$$\frac{D}{H} \times V = \frac{250 \text{ mg}}{125 \text{ mg}} \times 5 \text{ cc} =$$

_____ cc will be given.

10

On the next page are some problems for reviewing this material. The formula may be used with any measurement system. When two different systems of measurement are involved, the D and the H must be in the same system to proceed with the calculation.

PRACTICE PROBLEMS

ORAL MEDICATIONS

(ANSWERS ON PAGE 50)

---

1. From dipyridamole (Persantine) 25 mg, give 50 mg.

2. From digoxin (Lanoxin) 0.25 mg, give 0.125 mg.

3. From propranolol hydrochloride (Inderal) 10 mg, give 40 mg.

4. You have sulfisoxazole (Gantrisin) tablets on hand, gr v. How will you give 1.0 g?

5. Give phenobarbital gr ss from tablets 15.0 mg.

6. From cephradine (Velosef) 250 mg capsules, give 500 mg.

7. From tetracycline $\dfrac{125 \text{ mg}}{5 \text{ cc}}$, give 375 mg.

8. How many tablets labeled 10.0 mg will be given to administer $\text{gr}\dfrac{1}{6}$?

9. From amoxicillin $\dfrac{250 \text{ mg}}{5 \text{ ml}}$ give gr xv.

ANSWERS TO PROBLEMS ON PAGE 49

ORAL MEDICATIONS

1. $\dfrac{D}{H} = \dfrac{50 \text{ mg}}{25 \text{ mg}}$ = 2 tablets of dipyridamole 25 mg will be used.

2. $\dfrac{D}{H} = \dfrac{0.125 \text{ mg}}{0.25 \text{ mg}} = \dfrac{1}{2}$ tablet of digoxin 0.25 is used.

3. $\dfrac{D}{H} = \dfrac{40 \text{ mg}}{10 \text{ mg}}$ = 4 tablets of propranolol hydrochloride 10 mg.

4. 1.0 g = gr xv

   $\dfrac{D}{H} = \dfrac{\text{gr } 15}{\text{gr } 5}$ = 3 tablets of sulfisoxazole gr v will be given.

5. gr ss = 30.0 mg

   $\dfrac{D}{H} = \dfrac{30.0 \text{ mg}}{15.0 \text{ mg}}$ = 2 tablets of phenobarbital 15.0 mg will be given.

6. $\dfrac{D}{H} = \dfrac{500 \text{ mg}}{250 \text{ mg}}$ = 2 tablets of cephradine hydrochloride 250 mg will be given.

7. $\dfrac{D}{H} \times V = \dfrac{375 \text{ mg}}{125 \text{ mg}} \times 5 \text{ cc} = 3 \times 5 \text{ cc} = 15 \text{ cc}$ will be given.

8. 10.0 mg = gr $\dfrac{1}{6}$

   Give one tablet of drug labeled 10.0 mg.

9. gr xv = 1.0 g = 1,000.0 mg

   $\dfrac{D}{H} \times V = \dfrac{1,000 \text{ mg}}{250 \text{ mg}} \times 5 \text{ ml} = 4 \times 5 \text{ ml} = 20 \text{ ml}$ will be given.

7

SYRINGES

Many medications are given parenterally, that is, by injection—subcutaneously, intramuscularly, or intradermally. Three types of syringes are used: tuberculin, insulin, and hypodermic. The syringe selected is determined by the route and the amount of drug to be given.

Insulin syringes are especially designed for use with U-100 insulin and are calibrated in 1-unit measures.

The tuberculin syringe is a narrow 1-ml syringe. It is calibrated in $\frac{1}{10}$- and $\frac{1}{100}$-ml units on one side and minims on the other side.

The hypodermic syringe comes in various sizes. The most commonly used size is a 3-ml syringe calibrated in $\frac{1}{10}$-ml increments on one side and minims on the other side.

In this chapter, you will learn which syringe is appropriate to use to administer a given drug.

---

1. The nurse selects a syringe to use depending on the quantity of solution to be given, the drug, the route, and the body size. To determine which syringe to use, the nurse must calculate the _____ of the solution.	quantity

2. The tuberculin syringe is a narrow 1-ml syringe. It is marked off in $\frac{1}{10}$ ml, $\frac{1}{100}$ ml, and minims. The tuberculin syringe is used for injections _____ than 1 ml.

less

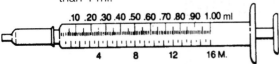

3. The insulin syringe is a narrow 1.0-ml or 0.5-ml syringe marked off in single units. It is used <u>only</u> for insulin that contains 100 units/ml. The insulin syringe would / <u>would</u> <u>not</u> be used for heparin.

would not

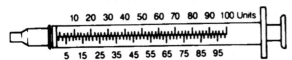

4. The hypodermic syringe most commonly used is a 3-ml syringe. It is marked off in $\frac{1}{10}$ ml and minims. The _____ syringe would be used for quantities of drug greater than 1 ml.

hypodermic

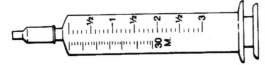

The hypodermic syringe also comes in sizes of 5 ml marked off in $\frac{1}{5}$ ml, 10 ml marked off in $\frac{1}{5}$ ml, 20 ml marked off in 1-ml increments, 30 ml marked off in increments of 1 ml, and 50 ml marked off in increments of 1 ml.

5. Needle gauges vary. The higher the gauge number, the smaller the needle. For instance, a 25-gauge needle is _____ than a 21-gauge needle.

smaller

6. The lengths of needles also vary, from $\frac{3}{8}$ inch to $1\frac{1}{2}$ inch. A 25-gauge needle, $\frac{1}{2}$ to $\frac{5}{8}$ inch long, is used for a subcutaneous injection since only the subcutaneous layer is to be penetrated.

To give a subcutaneous injection, the nurse would use a _____ gauge, _____-inch needle.

25

$\frac{1}{2}$ or $\frac{5}{8}$

7. The tuberculin syringe has a 26- to 27-gauge needle $\frac{3}{8}$ to $\frac{5}{8}$ inch long for intradermal injections. The tuberculin syringe with its small needle would be used for _____ injections.

The hypodermic syringe has a needle of 18 to 22 gauge and is 1 to $1\frac{1}{2}$ inches in length. The needle size to be used is determined by the viscosity of the medication and the size of the patient.

intradermal

8. If a medication for intramuscular injection is drawn up in a tuberculin syringe because it is a quantity less than 1 ml, the needle must be changed. If it is for an intramuscular injection, the needle would be changed to a(n) _____-gauge, _____-inch needle.

18- to 22   1 to $1\frac{1}{2}$

9. Some medications come in prefilled cartridges which are inserted into special holders in order to be able to inject them. These are called Tubex or Carpuject. If these are used, read the manufacturer's directions.

10. Now let's determine which syringe to use for the following orders.

Heparin 5,000 units SC is ordered. The vial contains 20,000 units per ml. How much would you need?

$$\frac{D}{H} \times V = \underline{\hspace{3cm}}$$

Fill in the proper numbers and complete the problem.

$$\frac{5,000 \text{ units}}{20,000 \text{ units}} \times 1 \text{ ml} = .25 \text{ ml}$$

11. In the preceeding problem, a(n)

_____ syringe would be used.

The needle must be changed to a(n)

_____-gauge, _____

inch needle to give a subcutaneous injection.

tuberculin

$25 \qquad \frac{1}{2} \text{ or } \frac{5}{8}$

12. The order reads 25 units Humulin N insulin SC in A.M. The vial contains Humulin N 100 units/ml. A(n)

_____ syringe would be used

and _____ units of insulin drawn into the syringe.

insulin

25

13. Hydroxyzine 75 mg IM is ordered. The vial reads 100 mg/2 ml. A(n) _____ syringe would be used and _____ ml drawn into the syringe.	3-ml hypodermic 1.5
14. Meperidine 50 mg IM is ordered. The vial contains 100 mg/ml. A(n) _____ syringe would be used and _____ ml given.	tuberculin (with the needle changed to 18- to 22- gauge, 1 to $1\frac{1}{2}$ inches long) .50 ml

Following are some practice problems. Decide the volume of medication to give, the type of syringe to use, and the needle gauge and length.

PRACTICE PROBLEMS

SYRINGES

(ANSWERS ON PAGE 56)

1. The order reads: "Meperidine 75 mg IM." The vial contains 100 mg/ml.

2. The order reads: "Atropine sulfate 0.4 mg IM." The vial contains 1 mg/ml.

3. The doctor ordered hydroxyzine hydrochloride 50 mg. The vial contains 50 mg/ml.

4. The order reads: "Humulin regular insulin 20 units SC." On hand is a vial with Humulin regular 100 units/ml.

5. The order reads: "Cimetidine 300 mg IM." The drug comes 300 mg/2 ml.

ANSWERS TO PROBLEMS ON PAGE 55

SYRINGES

---

1. $\dfrac{D}{H} \times V = \dfrac{75\text{ mg}}{100\text{ mg}} \times 1\text{ ml} = \dfrac{3}{4} \times 1\text{ ml} = \dfrac{3}{4}\text{ ml}$

   Use a tuberculin syringe and change the needle to an 18- to 22-gauge needle, 1 to $1\frac{1}{2}$ inches long.

2. $\dfrac{D}{H} \times V = \dfrac{0.4\text{ mg}}{1\text{ mg}} \times 1\text{ ml} = 0.4\text{ ml}$

   Use a tuberculin syringe and change the needle to an 18- to 22-gauge needle, 1 to $1\frac{1}{2}$ inches long.

3. $\dfrac{D}{H} \times V = \dfrac{50\text{ mg}}{50\text{ mg}} \times 1\text{ ml} = 1\text{ ml}$

   Use a 3-ml hypodermic syringe with an 18- to 22-gauge needle, 1 to $1\frac{1}{2}$ inches long.

4. Use an insulin syringe and draw 20 units of insulin.

5. Use a 3-ml hypodermic syringe and draw 2 ml of medication.

8

INJECTABLE LIQUIDS

There are many drugs that may be stored safely in liquid form. These drugs are packaged in ampules (single-dose) or vials (single-dose or multiple-dose) and are labeled according to the amount of the drug in the ampule or in a fractional part of the vial; for example, meperidine hydrochloride 50 mg (ampule), or meperidine hydrochloride 50 mg/cc (multi-dose vial). These drugs are administered parenterally.

Should the doctor's order for the medication and the drug that is available differ in dosage, you will use the formula discussed in this chapter to determine the quantity of solution to be given. Remember, as in working all dosage problems, two systems of weights and measures cannot be used in one problem without first converting the units to a common system.

---

1. Drugs for hypodermic injection are often kept in solutions of various strengths. These drugs are packaged in <u>ampules</u> or <u>vials</u>. An ampule holds a single dose, while a vial holds more than one dose. If you have four doses packaged together, this is called a

   _____.

   vial

---

2. The container will be labeled as to the <u>amount</u> <u>of</u> <u>drug</u> in the ampule or the fractional part of the vial. A vial labeled gr $\frac{1}{4}$ per cc would contain gr $\frac{1}{4}$ of the drug in each _____ of solution.

   cc

---

3. When the prescribed dose and the label on the ampule are the same, the nurse will use _____ of the ampule.

all

4. You are to give 50.0 mg of the drug. When the vial is labeled 50.0 mg per cc the nurse will withdraw _____ cc of solution from the vial.

1.0

5. When the prescribed dose differs from the label, the nurse must determine how much of the _____ must be used to give the prescribed dose.

solution

6. To determine the amount of solution required, use the following formula:

$$\frac{D}{H} \times V = x$$

In this formula:

D stands for _____

desired dose

H stands for _____

dose on hand

V stands for the volume on hand

x stands for the desired volume.

7. Example:

The vial is labeled "Morphine sulfate:

minims xv $= $ gr $\frac{1}{8}$."

Give gr $\frac{1}{6}$.

$$\frac{D}{H} \times V = x$$

$$\frac{gr\ 1/6}{gr\ 1/8} \times M.\ 15 = x$$

$$(\frac{1}{6} \times \frac{8}{1}) \times M.\ 15 =$$

$$(\frac{8}{6}) \times M.\ 15 =$$

$$1.33 \times M.\ 15 =$$

$$x = \underline{\hspace{3cm}}$$

20 minims of solution will be needed to give

morphine sulfate gr $\frac{1}{6}$.

(The answer is rounded from 19.9 to 20.)

---

8. Example:

The vial is labeled "Prochlorperazine: 5.0 mg per ml."

How will you give 8.0 mg of the drug?

$$\frac{D}{H} \times V = x$$

$$\frac{8.0\ mg}{?} \times \underline{\hspace{1.5cm}?\hspace{1.5cm}} = x$$

5.0 mg   1.0 ml

---

9. $\frac{8.0\ mg}{5.0\ mg} \times 1.0\ ml =$

Finish the calculation and label the answer.

$1.6 \times 1\ ml = 1.6\ ml$ of prochlorperazine will be needed to give 8.0 mg.

If you feel that you understand the use of this formula, continue to the following practice problems. If you are not sure of yourself, go back to frame 1 of this section and try again.

PRACTICE PROBLEMS

INJECTABLE LIQUIDS

(ANSWERS ON PAGES 62–63)

---

1. From a streptomycin solution containing 500.0 mg in 1.0 cc, give 400.0 mg.

2. The vial on hand is labeled: "Morphine sulfate: Minims xxx = gr $\frac{1}{8}$." Give gr $\frac{1}{24}$ of morphine sulfate.

3. From a cortisone acetate solution containing 25.0 mg in 1.0 cc, give 90.0 mg.

4. The stock solution is labeled: "Meperidine: 1.0 cc = 50.0 mg." Give 75.0 mg of meperidine.

5. From scopolamine 0.4 mg per ml, give gr $\frac{1}{300}$.

6. Give chlorpromazine 0.050 g from solution labeled 25.0 mg per ml.

7. From digitoxin 0.2 mg per cc, give 0.3 mg.

8. From hydroxyzine 100 mg per 2 cc, give 50 mg.

ANSWERS TO PROBLEMS ON PAGE 61
INJECTABLE LIQUIDS

---

1. $\dfrac{D}{H} \times V = x$

$\dfrac{400.0 \text{ mg}}{500.0 \text{ mg}} \times 1.0 \text{ cc} = x$

$0.8 \times 1.0 \text{ cc} = x$

$x = 0.8$ cc of the streptomycin solution 500.0 mg in 1.0 cc is needed to give streptomycin 400.0 mg.

2. $\dfrac{D}{H} \times V = x$

$\dfrac{\text{gr } 1/24}{\text{gr } 1/8} \times 30 \text{ minims} = x$

$(\dfrac{1}{24} \times \dfrac{8}{1}) \times 30 \text{ minims} = x$

$\dfrac{8}{24} \times 30 \text{ minims} = x$

$x = .33 \times 30 \text{ minims} = 9.9 \text{ minims (rounded off to 10)}$

$x = 10$ minims of the morphine sulfate solution M. xxx $=$ gr $\dfrac{1}{8}$ is needed to give morphine sulfate gr $\dfrac{1}{24}$.

3. $\dfrac{D}{H} \times V = x$

$\dfrac{90.0 \text{ mg}}{25.0 \text{ mg}} \times 1.0 \text{ cc} = x$

$3.6 \times 1.0 \text{ cc} = x$

$x = 3.6$ cc of the cortisone acetate solution 25.0 mg per 1.0 cc would be used (given IM because of the volume) in order to give cortisone acetate 90.0 mg.

4. $\dfrac{D}{H} \times V = x$

$\dfrac{75.0 \text{ mg}}{50.0 \text{ mg}} \times 1.0 \text{ cc} = x$

$1.5 \times 1.0 \text{ cc} = x$

$x = 1.5$ cc meperidine solution 50.0 mg per 1.0 cc will be used in order to give meperidine 75.0 mg (IM).

5. 0.4 mg $=$ gr $\dfrac{1}{150}$

$$\dfrac{D}{H} \times V = x$$

$$\dfrac{\text{gr } 1/300}{\text{gr } 1/150} \times 1.0 \text{ ml} = x$$

$$(\dfrac{1}{300} \times \dfrac{150}{1}) \times 1.0 \text{ ml} = x$$

$$\dfrac{150}{300} \times 1.0 \text{ ml} = x$$

$$0.5 \times 1.0 \text{ ml} = x$$

$x = 0.5$ ml of scopolamine solution labeled 0.4 mg/ml is needed to give scopolamine gr $\dfrac{1}{300}$.

6. 0.050 g $=$ 50.0 mg

$$\dfrac{D}{H} \times V = x$$

$$\dfrac{50.0 \text{ mg}}{25.0 \text{ mg}} \times 1.0 \text{ ml} = x$$

$$2 \times 1.0 \text{ ml} = x$$

$x = 2.0$ ml of the chlorpromazine solution labeled 25.0 mg/ml is needed to give chlorpromazine 0.050 g.

7. $\dfrac{D}{H} \times V = x$

$$\dfrac{0.3 \text{ mg}}{0.2 \text{ mg}} \times 1.0 \text{ cc} = x$$

$$1.5 \times 1.0 \text{ cc} = x$$

$x = 1.5$ cc of digitoxin solution labeled 0.2 mg/cc would be needed to give digitoxin 0.3 mg.

8. $\dfrac{D}{H} \times V = x$

$$\dfrac{50 \text{ mg}}{100 \text{ mg}} \times 2 \text{ cc} = x$$

$$0.5 \times 2 \text{ cc} = x$$

$x = 1$ cc of hydroxyzine solution labeled 100 mg per 2 cc would be needed to give hydroxyzine 50 mg.

9

DRUGS MEASURED IN UNITS

The strength of certain medications is measured in units. A unit is a specifically defined amount of anything subject to measurement. The unit is defined for each drug and there is no relationship between the strength of a unit of one drug and a unit of another drug. A unit of heparin cannot be compared to a unit of penicillin. It is also important to note that cubic centimeters and units are not interchangeable.

Insulin is an example of a medication that is measured in units. It is supplied in vials with 100 units per ml. The least complicated and most accurate way to measure insulin is to use an insulin syringe. This is a special 1.0-ml syringe calibrated to measure units rather than cubic centimeters and minims.

When you do not have an insulin syringe to give insulin, you may measure the dose by using a tuberculin syringe or an ordinary 3.0-ml hypodermic syringe. The quantity of insulin to be given is calculated by using the formula presented in this chapter and is measured in minims or cubic centimeters.

Tetanus antitoxin is another drug measured in units.

The formula (which is the same basic formula you have used before) may be used to calculate the dose of any drug which is measured in units.

---

1. Many biologicals are supplied in vials containing a specified number of units per cubic centimeter of the solution. A vial labeled 1,500 units per cc would contain _____ units of the drug in each cc of the solution.	1,500

---

2. The potency of the unit of each product is defined by the United States Pharmacopeia. The unit may also be called a U.S.P. _____.

unit

---

3. These drugs are ordered by the physician according to the number of _____ to be given.

units

---

4. When the vial is labeled 1,500 U.S.P. units (or 1,500 units) per cc, the nurse will withdraw _____ cc of solution to give 1,500 units.

1.0

---

5. When the prescribed dose differs from what is on hand, it is the nurse's responsibility to correctly calculate how much of the _____ must be given.

solution

---

6. Again use the basic formula:

$$\frac{\text{Desired dose (D)}}{\text{On-hand dose (H)}} \times V \text{ (Volume)}$$

Example:
The order is for 4,500 units of tetanus antitoxin. The label on the vial is "Tetanus Antitoxin: 1,500 units per milliliter." How much solution will be needed?

We will work together step by step:

$$\frac{D}{H} \times V = \frac{4,500 \text{ units}}{?} \times 1 \text{ ml}$$

1,500

7. $\dfrac{D}{H} \times V = \dfrac{4{,}500 \text{ ml}}{1{,}500 \text{ units per ml}} \times 1 \text{ ml}$

$\dfrac{45}{15} \times 1 \text{ ml} = $ _____ of tetanus antitoxin solution containing 1,500 units per ml will be needed to give 4,500 units of tetanus antitoxin.

3.0 ml

---

8. Example:
Using a penicillin solution containing 100,000 units in 1.0 cc, give 40,000 units of the drug.

$\dfrac{D}{H} \times V = $ _____

Substitute values and complete calculations. Label answer.

$\dfrac{40{,}000 \text{ units}}{100{,}000 \text{ units}} \times 1 \text{ cc} =$

$\dfrac{4}{10} \times 1 \text{ cc} = 0.4 \text{ cc of}$ penicillin solution containing 100,000 units in 1.0 cc will be needed to give 40,000 units of penicillin.

---

9. Example:
The order is for 25 units of Humulin N insulin. The label on the vial reads: "Humulin N: 100 units/cc."
How many cc are needed?

$\dfrac{D}{H} \times V = $ _____

$\dfrac{25 \text{ units}}{100 \text{ units}} \times 1 \text{ cc} =$

$.25 \times 1 \text{ cc} = .25 \text{ cc of}$ Humulin N will be needed to give 25 units.

10. Example:

The order is for 7,500 units of heparin sodium. The label reads: "Heparin sodium: 5,000 units/ml."

How many ml are needed?

$$\frac{D}{H} \times V = \underline{\hspace{3cm}}$$

$$\frac{7,500 \text{ units}}{5,000 \text{ units}} \times 1 \text{ ml} =$$

$$\frac{75}{50} \times 1 \text{ ml} = 1.5 \text{ ml will}$$

be needed to give 7,500 units heparin sodium.

Here are some practice problems.

PRACTICE PROBLEMS

DRUGS MEASURED IN UNITS

(ANSWERS ON PAGE 68)

1. From a vial labeled: "Heparin sodium: 20,000 units per ml," give 5,000 units of heparin sodium.

2. Give 50,000 units of sodium penicillin G from a multi-dose vial in which 10.0 ml contains 1,000,000 units.

3. Give penicillin 600,000 units from a solution labeled 3,000,000 units per 5.0 ml.

4. From penicillin 5,000,000 units per 10.0 cc, give penicillin 400,000 units.

5. How many minims of regular insulin U-100 will be needed to give 60 units?

6. How many cc of NPH insulin 100 units/cc will be needed to give 45 units?

7. From a vial labeled: "Heparin sodium: 5,000 units per ml," give 3,000 units.

ANSWERS TO PROBLEMS ON PAGE 67

DRUGS MEASURED IN UNITS

1. $\dfrac{D}{H} \times V = \dfrac{5,000 \text{ units}}{20,000 \text{ units}} \times 1 \text{ ml} =$

    $= 0.25$ ml of heparin sodium solution containing 20,000 units per ml will be needed to give 5,000 units of heparin sodium.

2. $\dfrac{D}{H} \times V = \dfrac{50,000 \text{ units}}{1,000,000 \text{ units}} \times 10 \text{ ml} =$

    $\dfrac{5}{100} \times 10 \text{ ml} = 0.5 \times 10 \text{ ml} = 0.5$ ml of penicillin G solution containing 1,000,000 units per 10.0 ml will be needed to give 50,000 units of penicillin G.

3. $\dfrac{D}{H} \times V = \dfrac{600,000 \text{ units}}{3,000,000 \text{ units}} \times 5 \text{ ml} =$

    $\dfrac{6}{30} \times 5 \text{ ml} = 0.2 \times 5 \text{ ml} = 1.0$ ml of penicillin solution labeled 3,000,000 units per 5.0 ml will be needed in order to give 600,000 units of penicillin.

4. $\dfrac{D}{H} \times V = \dfrac{400,000 \text{ units}}{5,000,000 \text{ units}} \times 10 \text{ cc} =$

    $\dfrac{4}{50} \times 10 \text{ cc} = 0.08 \times 10 \text{ cc} = 0.8$ cc penicillin solution containing 5,000,000 units per 10.0 cc will be needed in order to give 400,000 units of penicillin.

5. $\dfrac{D}{H} \times V = \dfrac{60 \text{ units}}{100 \text{ units}} \times 1 \text{ cc} = \dfrac{6}{10} \times 1 \text{ cc} = 0.6 \text{ cc}$

To change cc to minims, multiply the number of cc by 15.

    $0.6/\text{cc} \times 15 = 9$ minims of regular insulin U-100 will be needed to give 60 units.

6. $\dfrac{D}{H} \times V = \dfrac{45 \text{ units}}{100 \text{ units}} \times 1 \text{ cc} = 0.45 \times 1 \text{ cc} = 0.45 \text{ cc}$

0.45 cc of NPH insulin must be measured to give 45 units.

7. $\dfrac{D}{H} \times V = \dfrac{3,000 \text{ units}}{5,000 \text{ units}} \times 1 \text{ ml} = \dfrac{3}{5} \times 1 \text{ ml} = 0.6 \text{ ml}$

0.6 ml of heparin sodium labeled 5,000 units/ml will be needed to give 3,000 units.

10

PREPARATION OF DRUGS
PACKAGED IN POWDERS AND TABLETS

Drugs that are unstable in solution may also be packaged in dry form in ampules or vials. When you are ready to use the drug, you will dissolve the dry drug in the correct diluent. Information concerning the correct diluent will be packaged with the drug or may be obtained from the pharmacist or from pharmacology books. When a multi-dose vial is used, the vial must be relabeled stating the amount of drug contained in each cubic centimeter of the fluid and the date the fluid was prepared.

The formula you will need to solve this type of problem is presented here. This formula will be used only when the amount of the drug does not increase the amount of the solution. When the drug increases the amount of the solution, specific directions as to the quantity of diluent will be packaged with the drug and must be followed explicitly.

---

1. Certain drugs come from the pharmacy in <u>dry</u> <u>powder</u> <u>form</u> in a vial. The vial may contain the quantity of drug required for a single injection or may contain enough medication for several

_____.

doses

---

2. In a single-dose vial the amount of diluent used is usually 1.0 to 2.0 cc. However, the nurse should check the accompanying literature to determine

the optimum _____ and kind of diluent for that particular preparation.

amount

---

3. To determine the amount of diluent needed, a proportion must be used. The proportion formula to determine the amount of diluent needed is:

$$\frac{\text{Desired units}}{\text{On-hand units}} = \frac{\text{Desired volume}}{x \text{ volume}}$$

x volume is the amount of diluent which will be added to the dry drug.

Example:
The label on a vial of powdered penicillin reads: "Penicillin: 1,000,000 U.S.P. units." The physician has ordered penicillin 100,000 units stat and b.i.d. How many cubic centimeters of diluent will be needed to produce a solution containing 100,000 units per cc?

Use the formula above:

$$\frac{DU}{HU} = \frac{V}{x}$$

Substitute values:

$$\frac{100,000 \text{ units}}{1,000,000 \text{ units}} = \frac{?}{x}$$

1.0 cc

---

4. $\dfrac{100,000 \text{ units}}{1,000,000 \text{ units}} = \dfrac{1.0 \text{ cc}}{x}$

100,000 : 1,000,000 : : 1.0 cc : x

100,000x = 1,000,000 cc

$$x = \underline{\hspace{2cm}}$$

10.0 cc of diluent will be needed to produce penicillin solution of 100,000 units/cc.

---

5. After the diluent has been added to the vial, the vial must be labeled as to the number of units in each

$\underline{\hspace{2cm}}$.

cc

6. Another example:
How much diluent will be needed to make a solution of 100,000 units per cc if the vial contains 2,000,000 units of dry drug?

$$\frac{DU}{HU} = \frac{V}{x}$$

$$\frac{?}{?} = \frac{1.0 \text{ cc}}{x}$$

100,000
2,000,000

---

7. $\dfrac{100,000 \text{ units}}{2,000,000 \text{ units}} = \dfrac{1.0 \text{ cc}}{x}$

100,000 : 2,000,000 :: 1.0 cc : x

100,000x = 2,000,000.0 cc

$x =$ _____

20.0 cc of diluent will be needed to make a solution of 100,000 units/cc

---

8. Some drugs may increase the volume of the solution. This formula can be used only when the volume of the dry drug does not increase the volume of

the _____ .

solution

---

9. When the dry drug increases the volume of the solution, specific instructions will be given by the manufacturer

for the _____ of diluent to use.

amount

10. Example:
Streptomycin sulfate for injection.
The vial contains 1.0 g of the dry drug.
Instructions: for 100 mg per cc, add
9.2 cc of diluent.

The nurse will add 9.2 cc of diluent to
the dry drug, which will give a total of
10.0 cc of solution where each cc will

contain _____ of the drug.

100.0 mg

On the next page are some practice problems.

PRACTICE PROBLEMS

DRUGS IN POWDERS AND TABLETS

(ANSWERS ON PAGE 74)

---

1. How much diluent will be required to prepare a solution of benzathine penicillin G of 500,000 units per cc when the vial contains 1,000,000 units of the dry drug?

2. Given a vial containing 750 units of a drug in dry form, how will you prepare a solution containing 150 units per cc?

3. How much diluent will be needed to give a solution of 25,000 units per cc if the vial contains 200,000 units of dry drug?

4. A vial of potassium penicillin G contains 2,000,000 units of the dry drug. How much diluent will be needed to make a solution that contains 400,000 units per cc?

ANSWERS TO PROBLEMS ON PAGE 73

DRUGS PACKAGED IN POWDERS AND TABLETS

---

1. $\dfrac{DU}{HU} = \dfrac{V}{x}$

$\dfrac{500,000 \text{ units}}{1,000,000 \text{ units}} = \dfrac{1.0 \text{ cc}}{x}$

$500,000 : 1,000,000 :: 1.0 \text{ cc} : x$

$500,000x = 1,000,000 \text{ cc}$

$\qquad x = 2.0$ cc diluent will be needed to prepare a solution of benzathine penicillin G 500,000 units per cc.

2. $\dfrac{DU}{HU} = \dfrac{V}{x}$

$\dfrac{150 \text{ units}}{750 \text{ units}} = \dfrac{1.0 \text{ cc}}{x}$

$150 : 750 :: 1.0 \text{ cc} : x$

$150x = 750.0 \text{ cc}$

$\qquad x = 5.0$ cc diluent will be needed to prepare a solution containing 150 units of drug per cc.

3. $\dfrac{DU}{HU} = \dfrac{V}{x}$

$\dfrac{25,000 \text{ units}}{200,000 \text{ units}} = \dfrac{1.0 \text{ cc}}{x}$

$25,000 : 200,000 :: 1.0 \text{ cc} : x$

$25,000x = 200,000.0 \text{ cc}$

$\qquad x = 8.0$ cc diluent will be needed to prepare a solution containing 25,000 units of drug per cc.

4. $\dfrac{DU}{HU} = \dfrac{V}{x}$

$\dfrac{400,000 \text{ units}}{2,000,000 \text{ units}} = \dfrac{1.0 \text{ cc}}{x}$

$400,000 : 2,000,000 :: 1.0 \text{ cc} : x$

$400,000x = 2,000,000.0 \text{ cc}$

$\qquad x = 5.0$ cc diluent will be needed to prepare a solution containing 400,000 units of potassium penicillin G per cc.

11

MIXING PARENTERAL
MEDICATIONS

Often, two drugs may be mixed in a syringe to decrease the frequency of injection. The drugs mixed must be compatible, that is, they must not form a precipitate.

Mixing of drugs is common practice when two types of insulin are ordered and when preoperative medications are ordered.

Always check compatibility with the pharmacist or with a drug compatibility chart. If the drugs form a precipitate when mixed, discard them and inject each drug separately.

In this chapter, you will learn how to mix two drugs together in a syringe.

---

1. It is possible for the nurse to mix more than one medication in the same syringe to inject into the patient. This can provide for patient comfort by <u>decreasing/increasing</u> the number of injections needed.

decreasing

---

2. The nurse must check to see that the two medications are compatible—in other words, that they don't react to form a precipitate. If a precipitate forms, the nurse _____ give the injection.

cannot

3. When mixing two medications, it is important that the nurse not contaminate the medication left in one vial with the other medication. If contamination occurs, the contaminated drug must be _____.

discarded

4. When withdrawing two drugs from two separate vials, draw air into a syringe in an amount equal to the solution being withdrawn into vial #1. Inject this air into _____ _____, being careful to keep the needle out of the medication.
Withdraw the needle and syringe from vial #1 without the medication.

vial 1

5. Draw air into the syringe equaling the amount of solution to be withdrawn from vial #2 and inject this air into

_____ _____.

vial 2

6. Withdraw the correct amount of solution from vial #2. Change the needle and insert the syringe with the new needle into vial #1. Withdraw the correct amount of solution and remove the needle and syringe from vial #1.

The syringe has a _____ of the medications from vials #1 and #2, but neither is contaminated.

mixture

7. If a multi-dose vial and a single-dose vial are used, withdraw the medication from the multi-dose vial first to prevent

_____.

contamination

8. Example:

The order reads: "Meperidine 50 mg IM, hydroxyzine 50 mg IM on call to O.R." Meperidine is packaged in a vial containing 100 mg/cc; hydroxyzine in a vial containing 50 mg/cc.

Fill in the blanks.

You will need _____ cc of meperidine and _____ cc of hydroxyzine.

$$\frac{D}{H} \times V = \frac{50 \text{ mg}}{100 \text{ mg}} \times 1 \text{ cc}$$

$$= 0.5 \text{ cc meperidine}$$

$$\frac{D}{H} \times V = \frac{50 \text{ mg}}{50 \text{ mg}} \times 1 \text{ cc}$$

$$= 1 \text{ cc hydroxyzine}$$

---

9. Use a _____ syringe and draw up _____ cc of air and inject into the meperidine vial.

3-ml hypodermic

0.5

---

10. _____ the needle and syringe from the meperidine vial.

Remove

---

11. Draw up 1 cc of air and inject into the _____ vial. Withdraw 1 cc of the medication and remove the needle and syringe from the hydroxyzine vial.

hydroxyzine

---

12. _____ the needle and place the needle and syringe into the meperidine vial.

Change

---

13. Withdraw 0.5 cc of meperidine to a total of _____ cc in the syringe.

1.5

---

14. Insulins vary in their duration of action. There are short-, intermediate-, and long-acting insulins. (Review in a pharmacology text.) Often, two insulins are ordered together. They can be mixed in the same _____ syringe.

insulin

15. If the order reads 10 U regular insulin (short acting) and 25 U NPH (intermediate acting) SC before breakfast, and you had 100 units/cc insulin on hand, these two would be mixed in the following way:

Draw 25 units of air into the syringe and inject 25 units of air into the

_____ vial. Withdraw the needle and syringe from the NPH insulin vial.

NPH

---

16. Draw 10 units of air into the syringe

and inject into the _____ insulin vial.

regular

---

17. Withdraw _____ units of regular insulin from the vial and remove the needle and syringe from the regular insulin vial.

10

---

18. _____ the needle.

Change

---

19. Insert the new needle and syringe into the NPH insulin vial and withdraw

_____ units to a total of 35 units of insulin in the syringe (a mixture of 25 units NPH and 10 units regular).

25

20. *Always inject air in the longer-acting insulin vial first. Withdraw the shorter-acting insulin first, then the longer-acting insulin. If the shorter-acting insulin is accidentally injected into the vial containing the longer-acting insulin, the shorter-acting insulin will be absorbed. The longer-acting insulin cannot be absorbed by the shorter-acting insulin.*

Example:
The order reads 5 U regular insulin and 30 U NPH insulin in A.M. On hand is insulin with 100 units/cc.
Fill in the blanks.

Draw _____ units of air into the insulin syringe.

30

---

21. Inject the air into the _____ insulin vial and _____ the needle and syringe from the vial.

NPH

remove

---

22. Draw 5 units of air into the syringe and inject into the _____ insulin vial.

regular

---

23. Withdraw _____ units of regular insulin.

5

---

24. Change the needle and insert the needle and syringe into the _____ insulin vial.

NPH

---

25. Withdraw _____ units of NPH to a total of _____ units of insulin.

30

35

Here are a few practice problems. Go through all the steps of mixing medications in a syringe. Determine the amount of solution to be used and the type of syringe needed. Then explain how to mix the solution in the syringe.

PRACTICE PROBLEMS

MIXING PARENTERAL MEDICATIONS

(ANSWERS ON PAGES 82–83)

1. Order reads: "Meperidine 75 mg IM; hydroxyzine 25 mg IM." Meperidine comes 100 mg/ml. Hydroxyzine comes 100 mg/2 ml.

2. Order reads: "Regular insulin 15 U, NPH insulin 35 U SC." On hand is regular insulin 100 U/ml and NPH insulin 100 U/ml.

3. Order reads: "Morphine sulfate 10 mg IM and atropine sulfate 0.4 mg IM." On hand is morphine sulfate 10 mg/ml and atropine sulfate 1 mg/ml.

4. Order reads: "Regular insulin 5 units SC, NPH insulin 42 units SC." On hand is regular insulin 100 U/ml and NPH insulin 100 U/ml.

ANSWERS TO PROBLEMS ON PAGE 81

MIXING PARENTERAL MEDICATIONS

---

1. Use a 3 cc hypodermic syringe.

Draw back $\frac{3}{4}$ ml (0.75 ml or M. 12). $\quad \frac{D}{H} = \frac{75 \text{ mg}}{100 \text{ mg/ml}} = \frac{3}{4}$ ml

Inject $\frac{3}{4}$ ml into the meperidine vial and remove the needle and syringe.

Draw back $\frac{1}{2}$ ml. $\quad \dfrac{D}{H} = \dfrac{x}{2 \text{ ml}} \quad \begin{array}{l} 25 \text{ mg} : 100 \text{ mg} : : x : 2 \text{ ml} \\ 50 \text{ ml} = 100x \\ \qquad x = \dfrac{1}{2} \text{ ml} \end{array}$

Insert the needle and syringe in the hydroxyzine vial and inject $\frac{1}{2}$ ml air.

Withdraw $\frac{1}{2}$ ml hydroxyzine and remove the needle and syringe.

Change the needle.

Insert the new needle and syringe into the meperidine vial and remove 0.75 ml of meperidine to a total of $1\frac{1}{4}$ ml of medication in the syringe.

2. Use an insulin syringe.

Inject 35 units of air into the NPH insulin vial.

Remove the needle and syringe from the NPH insulin vial.

Inject 15 units of air into the regular insulin vial.

Remove 15 units of regular insulin and remove the needle and syringe from the regular insulin vial.

Change the needle.

Insert the new needle and syringe into the NPH insulin vial and remove 35 units to a total of 50 units of insulin mixed in the syringe.

3. Use a 3 cc hypodermic syringe.

Draw back 1 ml. $\dfrac{D}{H} = \dfrac{10 \text{ mg}}{10 \text{ mg/ml}} = 1$ ml

Inject 1 ml of air into the morphine sulfate vial and remove the needle and syringe.

Draw back 0.4 ml. $\dfrac{D}{H} = \dfrac{0.4 \text{ mg}}{1.0 \text{ mg/ml}} = 0.4$ ml

Insert the needle and syringe in the atropine sulfate vial.

Inject 0.4 ml of air into the atropine sulfate vial.

Withdraw 0.4 ml of atropine sulfate and remove the needle and syringe.

Change the needle.

Insert the new needle and syringe into the morphine sulfate vial and remove 10 mg (1 ml) to a total of 1.4 ml medication in the syringe.

4. Use an insulin syringe.

Inject 42 units of air into the NPH insulin vial.

Remove the needle and syringe from the NPH insulin vial.

Inject 5 units of air into the regular insulin vial.

Remove 5 units of regular insulin and remove the needle and syringe from the regular insulin vial.

Change the needle.

Insert the new needle and syringe into the NPH insulin vial and remove 42 units of NPH insulin to a total of 47 units.

12

PREPARATION OF SOLUTIONS

In giving nursing care, you may need to prepare a solution or to teach someone else how to do it. Solutions are commonly used for such purposes as irrigations or soaks and, depending on the situation, may be sterile or unsterile. A solution is a liquid containing a dissolved substance. It is made by dissolving one or more substances in a liquid (the solvent). These substances (solutes) may be in the form of a gas, a liquid, or a solid and may be the pure drug or the drug in a concentrated solution.

The strength of the solution is expressed in percentage or as a ratio. Percentage indicates the amount of the drug present in 100 parts of the solution. It is a fraction, the numerator of which is expressed, and the denominator understood to be 100; for example, 25 percent is 25/100. Ratio is another way of indicating the relationship between the amount of the drug and the amount of the solution; for example, a 1:10 solution contains one part of the pure drug in ten parts of solution. Ratio and percentage really mean the same thing. For instance, a 25 percent solution also can be expressed as a 1:4 solution. It is important to remember when working problems in percentage and ratio that all measurements must be kept in the same system.

---

1. When caring for patients, the nurse often will be called on to prepare a liquid or solution for irrigations, soaks, or other treatments. A liquid, homogeneous mixture consisting of two or more components is called a

_____.

solution

---

2. In most common solutions, one of the components is a liquid in which the other component is dissolved. This liquid portion is referred to as the solvent, and the component which is

_____ in it is known as the solute. The solute may be either solid or liquid.

dissolved

3. The most commonly used solvent is water. In a sodium chloride solution,

the solvent would be _____.

water

4. The solute in a sodium chloride solution would be _____. To make a physiologic saline solution, two teaspoons of table salt are dissolved in 1,000 ml of water.

sodium chloride

5. For a solution that need not be sterile (as a mouth wash), ordinary tap water is the _____ most frequently used.

solvent

6. To make a sterile solution (for use on a wound) the most common solvent would be _____ _____.

sterile water

7. Solutions are made from pure drugs, tablets, or stock solutions. A pure drug is an unadulterated substance in solid or liquid form. Expressed in percentage, a pure drug is _____.

100%

8. Tablets containing a known quantity of the pure drug may be used to make a solution. The _____ is essentially a preparation of the pure drug.

tablet

9. A stock solution is a relatively strong solution from which a weaker solution can be made. Stock solutions are usually _____ to make a weaker solution.

diluted

10. The strength of a solution may be expressed by percentage or ratio.
Percentage indicates:
(a) the number of grains of the drug in 100 grains
(b) the number of cc of the drug in 100.0 cc of the solution.
Thus, a 1% solution of peroxide contains 1.0 cc of peroxide in _____ solution. (Peroxide is a liquid.)

100.0 cc

11. In 200.0 cc of a 1% solution of peroxide, there are _____ of the pure drug.

2.0 cc

12. Ratio (when used with solutions) denotes the relative amounts of solute and solvent. Here, the metric system is almost invariably used. Thus: 1:1,000 indicates 1.0 g or 1.0 cc of pure drug in each 1,000.0 cc of solution.
2:1,000 therefore indicates 2.0 g (or 2.0 cc) of _____ _____ in 1,000.0 cc of solution.

pure drug

13. A solution labeled 1.0 ml:1,000 ml contains _____ solute in _____ solution.

1.0 ml   1,000 ml

14. Now, let's work some problems in which the strength of the solution is expressed in percentage.

The formula to be used is:

$$\frac{\text{Desired}}{\text{On-hand}} = \frac{\text{quantity of solute } (x)}{\text{quantity of solution } (V)}$$

or

$$\frac{D}{H} = \frac{x}{V}$$

Example:

How many cc of pure drug will be needed to prepare one liter of a 40% solution? How will you prepare the solution?

$$\frac{D}{H} = \frac{x}{V}$$

Substitute known values:

$$\frac{40\%}{?} = \frac{x}{1,000.0 \text{ cc } (1.0 \text{ liter})}$$

100%

15. $\dfrac{40\%}{100\%} = \dfrac{x}{?}$

1,000.0 cc

16. $100x = 40,000.0$ cc

$x =$ _____

400.0 cc of pure drug will be needed

17. To prepare the 40% solution of drug, place the 400.0 cc of pure drug in a container and add water to make

_____.

1,000.0 cc

18. Example:
Prepare 250.0 cc of a 1% neomycin sulfate solution. How much neomycin sulfate will be needed? How will you prepare the solution?

Use the formula:

$$\frac{D}{H} = \frac{x}{V}$$

$$\frac{1\%}{100\%} = \frac{?}{?}$$

$$\frac{x}{250.0 \text{ cc}}$$

19. $\dfrac{1\%}{100\%} = \dfrac{x}{250.0 \text{ cc}}$

Finish calculations and label answer.

$100x = 250.0 \text{ cc}$

$x = 2.5$ cc of neomycin sulfate will be needed. To this amount of drug add water to make 250.0 cc of solution. This is a 1% solution.

20. One more example:

5.0 g of boric acid for solution, sterile, is dispensed. How much 5% solution can be made from one vial?

Note: In this problem, the amount of solute is known rather than the amount of solution to be made.

The same basic formula is used:

$$\frac{D}{H} = \frac{V \text{ (quantity of solute)}}{x \text{ (quantity of solution)}}$$

$$\frac{5\%}{100\%} = \frac{5.0 \text{ g or cc}}{x}$$

Finish calculations and label answer.

$5x = 500.0 \text{ cc}$
$x = 100.0 \text{ cc}$
It is stated in the volume unit rather than solid unit. The 5.0 g of boric acid is dissolved in 100.0 cc of sterile water—100.0 cc of a 5% boric acid solution.

21. When the strength of the solution is expressed in ratio, this formula will be used:

$$\frac{\text{Desired Ratio}}{\text{On-hand Ratio}} = \frac{\text{quantity of solute}}{\text{quantity of solution}}$$

or

$$\frac{D}{H} = \frac{?}{?}$$

$$\frac{x}{V}$$

22. Example:

How much solute will be needed to make 2,000.0 ml of a 1:5,000 sodium bicarbonate solution from a 1:1,000 solution?

$$\frac{D}{H} = \frac{x}{V}$$

$$\frac{1:5,000}{1:1,000} = \frac{?}{?}$$

$$\frac{x}{2,000.0 \text{ ml}}$$

23. $\dfrac{1/5,000}{1/1,000} = \dfrac{x}{2,000.0 \text{ ml}}$

$\dfrac{1}{1,000x} = 2,000.0 \text{ ml} \times \dfrac{1}{5,000}$

$x = \underline{\hspace{2cm}}$

Finish calculations and label answer.

$x = \dfrac{2}{5} \text{ ml} \div \dfrac{1}{1,000}$

$x = 400.0 \text{ ml of the } \dfrac{1}{1,000}$

sodium bicarbonate solution will be needed. (Note: Here, the problem asks only how much drug will be needed.)

24. Example:
How will you prepare one quart of 1:20 solution of boric acid from the crystals?

$\dfrac{D}{H} = \dfrac{x}{V}$

$\dfrac{1/20}{1/1} = \dfrac{x}{1,000.0 \text{ cc}}$

(This is the equivalent of one quart.)

$1x = 1,000.0 \text{ cc} \times \dfrac{1}{20}$

$x = \underline{\hspace{2cm}}$ of boric acid crystals will be needed. Add water to make

$\underline{\hspace{2cm}}$ solution. You now have one quart of 1:20 solution of boric acid.

50g

1,000.0 cc (1 quart)
(Note: This problem asks how you will prepare the solution.)

On the next page are some practice problems. When solving these problems, remember to put all measurements into the same system.

PRACTICE PROBLEMS

SOLUTIONS

(ANSWERS ON PAGES 92–95)

---

1. From a 3% hydrogen peroxide solution, how will you prepare one ounce of a 1% solution?

2. How will you make one quart of a 10% solution of neomycin sulfate?

3. How much hydrochloric acid will be needed to make two liters of a 2% solution?

4. How many cc of 0.02% potassium permanganate solution can be made from 0.3 g of potassium permanganate crystals?

5. How much 0.25% sodium hypochlorite solution can be made from 250.0 cc of a 1% sodium hypochlorite solution?

6. How will you make 200.0 ml of a 1:40 acetic acid solution from a 1:20 acetic acid solution?

7. How much 75% solution of alcohol will be required to make one pint of a 1:2 alcohol solution?

8. Make one gallon of 5% boric acid solution from a 1:5 boric acid solution.

9. Prepare 1,000.0 cc of 1:5,000 solution of potassium permanganate from a 1:500 solution.

10. Prepare 50.0 cc of a 10% solution of magnesium sulfate from a 1:2 magnesium sulfate solution.

11. How much stock solution of benzalkonium chloride 1:1,000 will be needed to make one liter of 1:10,000 solution?

12. How many 5-grain tablets are needed to prepare two liters of 1:6,000 potassium permanganate solution?

13. How will you prepare 300.0 cc of 1:20,000 solution from a silver nitrate solution 1:1,000?

ANSWERS TO PROBLEMS ON PAGE 91

SOLUTIONS

1. $\dfrac{D}{H} = \dfrac{x}{V}$

$\dfrac{1\%}{3\%} = \dfrac{x}{30.0 \text{ cc}}$ (equivalent of 1 fluidounce)

$3x = 30.0$ cc
   $x = 10.0$ cc of 3% hydrogen peroxide solution will be needed. Add water to make 30.0 cc (1 fluidounce). You now have 1 ounce of 1% hydrogen peroxide solution.

2. $\dfrac{D}{H} = \dfrac{x}{V}$

$\dfrac{10\%}{100\%} = \dfrac{x}{1,000.0 \text{ cc}}$ (equivalent of 1 quart)

$100x = 10,000.0$ cc
   $x = 100.0$ cc neomycin sulfate will be needed. Add water to make 1,000 cc (1 quart). You now have 1 quart of 10% neomycin sulfate solution.

3. $\dfrac{D}{H} = \dfrac{x}{V}$

$\dfrac{2\%}{100\%} = \dfrac{x}{2,000.0 \text{ cc}}$

$100x = 4,000.0$ cc
   $x = 40.0$ cc of hydrochloric acid will be needed. Add water to make 2,000.0 cc. You now have 2 liters of 2% hydrochloric acid solution.

4. 1.0 g = 1.0 cc   0.3 g = 0.3 cc

$$\frac{D}{H} = \frac{x}{V}$$

$$\frac{0.02\%}{100\%} = \frac{0.3 \text{ cc}}{x}$$

$0.02x = 30.0$ cc
    $x = 1,500.0$ cc of 0.02% potassium permanganate solution can be
        made from 0.3 g potassium permanganate.

5. $\dfrac{D}{H} = \dfrac{V}{x}$

$$\frac{0.25\%}{1\%} = \frac{250.0 \text{ cc}}{x}$$

$0.25x = 250.0$ cc
    $x = 1,000.0$ cc of 0.25% sodium hypochlorite solution can be made
        from 250.0 cc of 1% sodium hypochlorite solution.

6. $\dfrac{D}{H} = \dfrac{x}{V}$

$$\frac{1/40}{1/20} = \frac{x}{200.0 \text{ ml}}$$

$$\frac{1}{20}x = 200.0 \text{ ml} \times \frac{1}{40}$$
    $x = 100.0$ ml of 1:20 acetic acid solution needed. Add water to make
        200.0 ml of 1:40 acetic acid solution.

7. Change 1:2 to the percent equivalent—50%
    $(1:2 = \dfrac{1}{2}$ $\dfrac{1}{2} \times 100 = 50\%)$

$$\frac{D}{H} = \frac{x}{V}$$

$$\frac{50\%}{75\%} = \frac{x}{500.0 \text{ cc}} \text{ (equivalent of 1 pint)}$$

$75x = 25,000.0$ cc
    $x = 333.33$ cc of 75% alcohol will be needed. (Round off to 333.0 cc.)
        Add water to make 500.0 cc. You now have 1 pint of 1:2 alcohol
        solution.

8. 1 gallon = 4,000.0 cc

Change 5% to its ratio equivalent 1:20

$(5\% = \dfrac{5}{100} = \dfrac{1}{20} = 1:20.$ Do you need to review this process?)

$$\dfrac{D}{H} = \dfrac{x}{V}$$

$$\dfrac{1/20}{1/5} = \dfrac{x}{4{,}000.0 \text{ cc}}$$

$$\dfrac{1}{5}x = 4{,}000.0 \text{ cc} \times \dfrac{1}{20}$$

$x = 1{,}000.0$ cc of 1:5 boric acid solution is needed to make 4,000.0 cc (1 gallon). You now have 1 gallon of 5% boric acid solution.

9. $\dfrac{D}{H} = \dfrac{x}{V}$

$$\dfrac{1/5{,}000}{1/500} = \dfrac{x}{1{,}000.0 \text{ cc}}$$

$$\dfrac{1}{500}x = 1{,}000.0 \text{ cc} \times \dfrac{1}{5{,}000}$$

$x = 100.0$ cc of $\dfrac{1}{500}$ potassium permanganate solution is needed.

Add water to make 1,000.0 cc. You now have 1,000.0 cc of 1:5,000 solution of potassium permanganate.

10. Change 10% to its ratio equivalent 1:10

$(10\% = \dfrac{10}{100} = \dfrac{1}{10} = 1:10)$

$$\dfrac{D}{H} = \dfrac{x}{V}$$

$$\dfrac{1/10}{1/2} = \dfrac{x}{50.0 \text{ cc}}$$

$$\dfrac{1}{2}x = 50.0 \text{ cc} \times \dfrac{1}{10}$$

$x = 10.0$ cc of 1:2 magnesium sulfate solution is needed. Add water to make 50.0 cc. You now have 50.0 cc of a 10% magnesium sulfate solution.

11. $\dfrac{D}{H} = \dfrac{x}{V}$

$$\dfrac{1/10,000}{1/1,000} = \dfrac{x}{1,000.0 \text{ cc}}$$

$$\dfrac{1}{1,000}x = 1,000.0 \text{ cc} \times \dfrac{1}{10,000}$$

$x = 100.0$ cc of 1:1,000 benzalkonium chloride solution will be needed.

12. gr 5 = 0.3 g

$$\dfrac{D}{H} = \dfrac{x}{V}$$

$$\dfrac{1/6,000}{1/1} = \dfrac{x}{2,000.0 \text{ cc (2 liters)}}$$

$$x = 2,000.0 \text{ cc} \times \dfrac{1}{6,000}$$

$x = 0.3$ g (Since weight unit is desired, pure drug will be needed.) Therefore:

$\dfrac{D}{H} = \dfrac{0.3 \text{ g}}{0.3 \text{ g}} =$ 1 potassium permanganate tablet 0.3 g or 1 potassium permanganate tablet gr 5 will be needed.

13. $\dfrac{D}{H} = \dfrac{x}{V}$

$$\dfrac{1/20,000}{1/1,000} = \dfrac{x}{300.0 \text{ cc}}$$

$$\dfrac{1}{1,000}x = 300.0 \text{ cc} \times \dfrac{1}{20,000}$$

$x = 15.0$ cc of 1:1,000 silver nitrate solution will be needed. Add water to make 300.0 cc. You now have 300.0 cc of 1:20,000 silver nitrate solution.

13

INTRAVENOUS MEDICATIONS

In your nursing practice you will frequently administer fluids and electrolyte solutions to your patients by intravenous infusion. Large hospitals may have special intravenous therapy teams with the function of starting infusions, while in a smaller hospital the staff nurse may have this responsibility. Regardless of who starts the infusion, each and every nurse who has contact with the patient shares the responsibility for the safe and therapeutic administration of any solution.

The purpose of this chapter is to help you develop the skills necessary to calculate proper flow rates and to determine the amount of fluid or drug the patient is receiving in a specific period of time.

1. When an order for <u>fluid administration</u> is written it should include the solution to be administered and the rate of administration. Usually the order will be written thus:

"1,000 cc D_5W q 8 hours IV" indicating that 1,000 cc of D_5W is to be infused

over a period of _____ hours.

8

2. To further simplify, determine the amount of fluid to be administered in one hour using the following formula:

Total amount ÷ Total time = amount to be administered in one hour.

In the above example: 1,000 cc ÷ 8 =

_____ cc administered in 1 hour.

125

3. Parenteral administration sets deliver fluids by drops (via a drip chamber) which vary in size.

The larger the size of the drop, the fewer the number of drops that will be needed to administer 1 cc. The smaller

the size of the drop, the _____ the number of drops that will be needed to administer 1 cc.

greater

4. Information on drop size is available from the manufacturer of the equipment, and should be indicated on the set. This is called the drop factor. Example: A set labeled with a drop factor

of 10 will need _____ drops to administer 1 cc of the solution.

10

5. A drop factor of 15 indicates the set will deliver 1 cc of fluid for every

_____ drops.

15

6. When the drop factor is known, the drops per minute necessary to administer a specific amount of fluid in a prescribed time period is easily calculated by using the following formula:

$$\text{Drops/min.} = \frac{\text{Total cc} \times \text{drop factor}}{\text{minutes}}$$

In the previous example, the number of cc to be administered IV in one hour was determined:

1,000 cc ÷ 8 = _____   125 cc per hour

---

7. Next, using a drop factor of 10, set up the formula:

$$\text{Drops/min.} = \frac{\text{Total cc} \times \text{drop factor}}{\text{minutes}}$$

$$x = \frac{125 \text{ cc} \times \underline{\quad ? \quad}}{60 \text{ minutes}}$$ 10

---

8. Solve for x.

$$x = \frac{125 \times 10}{60}$$

$$x = \frac{125}{6}$$

x = 20.8 or
  = 21 drops/min. to
deliver 125 cc in 1 hour
or 1,000 cc in 8 hours.

---

9. Try another problem. The order reads "Administer by IV 500 cc D₅W in 4 hours." A check of your equipment indicates the drop factor to be 10. Now you have all the information necessary to determine the flow rate, or the

_____ _____ _____   number of drops
                                                          per minute
_____ _____.

10. Take it step by step. First, determine the amount of solution to be delivered in one hour:

Total amount ÷ Total time = amount per minute.

or

500 cc ÷ 4 hours = _____.

125 cc

---

11. The drop factor given above is

_____.

10

---

12. The time (in minutes) is _____.

60

---

13. Using the flow rate formula

Drops/min. =
$$\frac{\text{Amount in cc} \times \text{drop factor}}{\text{time in minutes}}$$

Substitute known values and solve for x.

$$x = \frac{125 \text{ cc} \times 10}{60 \text{ min.}}$$

$x = 125 \div 6$

$x = 20.8$ or 21 drops/min. to administer 125 cc fluid in 1 hour or 500 cc in 4 hours.

---

14. Order: "200 cc 0.9 NaCl IV in 2 hours." The drop factor is 15. What is the flow rate per minute?

200 cc ÷ 2 hours
= 100 cc in 1 hour

$$x = \frac{100 \times 15}{60}$$

$x = 100 \div 4$

$x = 25$ drops/min. to administer 100 cc 0.9 NaCl in 1 hour or 200 cc in 2 hours.

15. It is frequently necessary to administer very small quantities of fluid over a period of time (for example, to infants or when very potent drugs are being given). To facilitate this, the flow is measured in microdrops per minute. Most of the sets used for this purpose have drop chambers which deliver 60 microdrops per cc. These sets are designated as Pedi-sets or Microdrip sets.

The flow rate for a Microdrip set is

_____.

60

16. Use the flow rate formula to implement the following order: "100 cc of 10% glucose in D_5W by intravenous to a 10-month-old over 4 hours."

100 cc in 4 hours = _____ in 1 hour.

25 cc

17. Using a Pedi-set, delivering 60 drops/ cc, substitute known values in the formula and solve for x.

Microdrops/min. =

$$\frac{\text{Total amount} \times \text{drop factor}}{\text{Time}}$$

$$x = \frac{25 \text{ cc} \times 60}{60 \text{ minutes}}$$

$x = 25$ microdrops/min. to deliver 25 cc in 1 hour or 100 cc in 4 hours.

18. Here is another order:
"Give 500 cc 0.45 NaCl by IV in 10 hours." The Microdrop set has a drop factor of 60.

You will regulate the set to run at

_____ microdrops/min.

500 cc ÷ 10
= 50 cc in one hour

$$x = \frac{50 \text{ cc} \times 60}{60 \text{ minutes}}$$

x = 50 microdrops/min. to administer 50 cc in one hour or 500 cc in 10 hours.

Easy, isn't it? If you did make an error, please go back to frame 6 and identify the error.

19. You may have noted in the above examples that when using a Pedi- or Micro-set delivering 60 drops/cc, the number of cc delivered each hour is equal to the number of drops per minute.

Therefore, when using a set that delivers 60 drops per cc you will not need to calculate the flow rate by the previous formula. Instead, consider:

Drops/min. = cc/hour

or

15 drops/min. = _____ cc/hour

15

REMEMBER: Before using this shortcut, be sure the set you are using delivers 60 drops/cc.

20. Sometimes, an IV medication is ordered to be infused by a dose and the nurse must calculate the flow rate. (To calculate the flow rate, a proportion must be used.)

For example, an order reads: "Heparin 2,000 units/hr from an IV solution of 20,000 units of heparin in 1,000 cc NSS."

How many ml/hr are to be infused?

$$\frac{20{,}000 \text{ units}}{\underline{\quad ? \quad} \text{ ml}} = \frac{2{,}000 \text{ units/hr}}{x \text{ ml}}$$

1,000

---

21. $1{,}000 \times 2{,}000 = \underline{\hspace{2cm}} x$

20,000

$2{,}000{,}000 = 20{,}000x$

$2{,}000{,}000 \div 20{,}000 = x \text{ ml/hr}$

$x = \underline{\hspace{2cm}} \text{ ml/hr}$

100

---

22. Another example is:
Pitocin is ordered to run at 0.02 units per minute from an IV solution of 10 units/1,000 ml PSS. How many ml/hr are to be infused?

The first thing that must be done is to convert units/min to units/hr.

$0.02 \text{ U/min} = \underline{\hspace{2cm}} \text{ U/hr}$

$0.02 \times 60 = 1.2$

---

23. $\dfrac{10 \text{ U}}{1{,}000 \text{ ml}} = \dfrac{1.2 \text{ U}}{x \text{ ml}}$

$1{,}200 = 10x$

$1{,}200 \div \underline{\hspace{2cm}} = x \text{ ml/hr}$

10

$x = \underline{\hspace{2cm}} \text{ ml/hr}$

120

24. It may also be necessary to calculate hourly doses of medication when the hourly volume to be infused has been ordered. IT IS THE RESPONSIBILITY OF THE NURSE TO KNOW THE DOSAGE OF THE MEDICATION BEING ADMINISTERED.

For example, an order reads: "IV 1,000 ml PSS with 20,000 units of heparin to infuse at 100 ml/hr."

To calculate the dose that the patient receives every hour, a proportion is used.

$$\frac{20,000 \text{ U}}{1,000 \text{ ml}} = \frac{x \text{ U}}{100 \text{ ml}}$$

$x = $ _____

2,000 U/hr

---

25. IV pumps and IV controllers are also available. These are used for IV medications that must be delivered at an exact rate at all times. These pumps or controllers would only be used if a

_____ *must* be given at a set rate. Examples are lidocaine, aminophylline, and heparin.

medication

Each manufacturer includes specific instructions with the machines. It is essential to acquaint yourself with the machine and the set-up before using it.

Some IV medications are given through sets that control the volume. These volume-control sets are called Buretrol, Soluset, Volutrol, Peditrol. The manufacturer provides detailed instructions (usually included in the package). Read the directions carefully before using.

Here are some practice problems.

PRACTICE PROBLEMS

INTRAVENOUS MEDICATIONS

(ANSWERS ON PAGES 106–107)

1. Give 800 cc lactated Ringer's solution IV in four hours using a drop factor of 10. What is the flow rate to be used?

2. Your postoperative hysterectomy client has an order for 2,500 cc D_5 in $\frac{1}{2}$ NSS to be given IV every 12 hours. Your IV set has a drop factor of 15. You will adjust the set to deliver _____ drops per minute.

3. Give 1,000 cc NSS by IV in 10 hours. The drop factor is 15. What is the flow rate?

4. Give an infant 120 cc physiologic saline IV in 6 hours. The drop factor is 60. What is the flow rate?

5. Your postcholecystectomy client is to receive 250 cc packed cells in 2 hours. The blood administration set states "6 drops per cc." The flow rate will be _____.

6. Heparin 2,500 units an hour from an IV solution of 20,000 units in 1,000 ml NSS. How many ml per hour are to be infused?

7. The order reads: 500 mg of aminophylline in 250 ml D_5/W to run at 10 ml/hr. What is the dose that the patient receives in 1 hour?

ANSWERS TO PROBLEMS ON PAGE 105

INTRAVENOUS MEDICATIONS

---

1. 800 cc ÷ 4 hours = 200 cc in 1 hour

$$\text{Flow rate} = \frac{\text{Total cc} \times \text{drop factor}}{\text{Time in minutes}}$$

$$x = \frac{200 \text{ cc} \times 10}{60}$$

$$x = 200 \div 6$$

$x = 33\frac{1}{3}$ or 33 drops/min. to administer 200 cc lactated Ringer's solution IV in 1 hour or 800 cc in 4 hours.

2. 2,500 cc ÷ 12 hours = 208 cc per 1 hour

$$\text{Flow rate} = \frac{\text{Total cc} \times \text{drop factor}}{\text{Time in minutes}}$$

$$x = \frac{208 \times 15}{60}$$

$$x = 208 \div 4$$

$x = 52$ drops/min. to administer 208 cc D_5 in $\frac{1}{2}$ NSS IV in 1 hour or 2,500 cc in 12 hours.

3. 1,000 cc ÷ 10 hours = 100 cc in 1 hour

$$x = \frac{100 \times 15}{60}$$

$$x = 100 \div 4$$

$x = 25$ drops/min. to administer 100 cc NSS by IV in 1 hour or 1,000 cc in 10 hours.

4. 120 cc ÷ 6 hours = 20 cc in 1 hour

$$x = \frac{20 \times 60}{60}$$

x = 20 drops/min. to administer 20 cc physiologic saline in 1 hour or 120 cc in 6 hours.

5. 250 cc ÷ 2 hours = 125 cc in 1 hour

$$x = \frac{125 \times 6}{60}$$

x = 12.5 or 13 drops/min. to administer 125 cc packed cells in 1 hour or 250 cc in 2 hours.

6. $\dfrac{20,000 \text{ U}}{1,000 \text{ ml}} = \dfrac{2,500 \text{ U}}{x \text{ ml}}$

2,500,000 = 20,000x

2,50~~0,000~~ ÷ 20,~~000~~ = x ml/hr

x = 125 ml/hr

7. $\dfrac{500 \text{ mg}}{250 \text{ ml}} = \dfrac{x \text{ mg}}{10 \text{ ml}}$

5,000 = 250x

5,000 ÷ 250 = x

x = 20 mg aminophylline in 1 hour.

14

MEDICATIONS FOR INFANTS
AND CHILDREN

Medications may be administered to infants and children by any of the routes used for adults. When administering medications to infants and children, the nurse will note that the amount of the drug given is always less than the usual adult dose. The amount to be given is calculated as a fractional part of the adult dose based on weight, age, or body surface area. While the physician will state the amount of drug he wishes the patient to have, it is important that the nurse be able to recognize an overdose, and it is the nurse's responsibility to ensure that an overdose is not given.

In this chapter you will learn how to use the four methods most commonly used to estimate the amount of a drug to be given to an infant or a child. You must remember that these are used as guides only, and that the physiologic and pathologic condition of the patient will also influence the amount of medication given. In the determination of drug dosage, an individual over 12 is considered an adult; an individual between 2 and 12 is considered a child; and an individual from birth to 24 months is considered an infant. The methods based on weight may also be used to determine the amount of a drug to be given to adults as well as to infants and children.

---

1. Nurses who work with infants and children will observe that the amount of drug ordered is less than the usual adult dose. You will always question an order for an infant or child which is

the _____ as the usual adult dose.

same

---

2. While the dose of the drug for an infant or child will be ordered by the physician, it is important that the nurse be able to recognize whether this dose is within safe _____.

limits (or range)

3. Several rules are used in current practice as guides to estimate the dose of drugs for infants and children. No one rule is completely satisfactory; therefore, these rules should be used only as a _____.

guide

4. The most accurate way to estimate the dose for an infant or child is by the use of the body surface area. The physician will probably use the _____ _____ _____ of the patient to determine the amount of the drug the patient should have.

body surface area

Note: Body surface area is determined by the use of a <u>nomogram</u>. This is a method infrequently used by the nurse; therefore, we refer you to the standard pediatrics textbook for information on the nomogram itself, its use, and the formulas involved.

5. Rules which the nurse may use as a guide to estimate the correct dose for an infant or child are those based on the age and weight of the patient. If the age of the patient is known, you may use a rule based on _____ to calculate the dose.

age

6. Young's Rule is based on the age of the child. To estimate the dose of a drug for a 7-year-old boy the nurse could use _____ _____.

Young's Rule

7. Young's Rule states:

$$\frac{\text{child's}}{\text{dose}} = \frac{\text{age (in years)}}{\text{age (in years)} + 12} \times \frac{\text{adult}}{\text{dose}}$$

Substitute the age of the boy in frame 6:

$$\frac{\text{child's}}{\text{dose}} = \frac{?}{? + 12} \times \frac{\text{adult}}{\text{dose}}$$

7 years
7 years

8. Now we will work some problems using Young's Rule.

Example:
If an adult receives meperidine (Demerol) 50.0 mg, how much Demerol would a 3-year-old child receive?

$$\frac{\text{child's}}{\text{dose}} = \frac{\text{age (in years)}}{\text{age (in years)} + 12} \times \frac{\text{adult}}{\text{dose}}$$

Substitute in Young's Rule:

$$\frac{\text{child's}}{\text{dose}} = \frac{?}{?} \times \frac{\text{adult}}{\text{dose}}$$

3 years
3 years + 12

9. $\dfrac{\text{child's}}{\text{dose}} = \dfrac{3 \text{ years}}{3 \text{ years} + 12} \times 50.0 \text{ mg}$

$x = \dfrac{3}{15} \times 50 \text{ mg}$

$x =$ _____

Finish calculations and label answer.

$x = \dfrac{1}{5} \times 50.0 \text{ mg}$

$x = 10.0$ mg of Demerol is this child's dose.

10. Example:

An adult is receiving 0.5 g streptomycin. How much streptomycin would a child of 4 years receive?

$$\frac{\text{child's}}{\text{dose}} = \frac{\text{age (in years)}}{\text{age (in years)} + 12} \times \frac{\text{adult}}{\text{dose}}$$

Substitute values and complete calculations. Be sure to label your answer.

$$x = \frac{4 \text{ years}}{4 \text{ years} + 12} \times 0.5 \text{ g}$$

$$x = \frac{4}{16} \times 0.5 \text{ g}$$

$$x = \frac{1}{4} \times 0.5 \text{ g}$$

$x = 0.125$ g streptomycin is this child's dose.

---

11. Fried's Rule (based on age) is used to estimate the dose of drugs for an infant. When the age of the infant is known the

nurse may use _____ _____.

Fried's Rule

---

12. Fried's Rule states:

$$\frac{\text{infant's}}{\text{dose}} = \frac{\text{age in months}}{150 \text{ months}} \times \frac{\text{adult}}{\text{dose}}$$

Note: 150 months here indicates $12\frac{1}{2}$ years (adult age).

Substitute in the formula for an infant of 15 months where the usual adult dose is gr 1.

$$\frac{\text{infant's}}{\text{dose}} = \frac{\text{age in months}}{150 \text{ months}} \times \frac{\text{adult}}{\text{dose}}$$

$$\frac{\text{infant's}}{\text{dose}} = \frac{}{150 \text{ months}} \times \frac{}{}$$

15 months   gr 1

13. Solve the following problem, again working step by step.

Example:
Determine the dosage of sulfisoxazole (Gantrisin) for a 15-month-old infant. Consider the adult dose of Gantrisin to be 0.5 g.

$$\frac{\text{infant's}}{\text{dose}} = \frac{\text{age in months}}{150 \text{ months}} \times \frac{\text{adult}}{\text{dose}}$$

Substitute values in Fried's Rule:

$$x = \frac{?}{?} \times \text{adult dose (0.5 g)}$$

$$\frac{15 \text{ months}}{150 \text{ months}}$$

---

14. $x = \dfrac{15 \text{ months}}{150 \text{ months}} \times 0.5 \text{ g}$

$x = $ _____

Complete calculations and be sure to label your answer.

$$\frac{15 \text{ months}}{150 \text{ months}} \times 0.5 \text{ g}$$

$$x = \frac{1}{10} \times 0.5 \text{ g}$$

$x = 0.05$ g of Gantrisin is this infant's dose.

---

15. Try another problem:

If an adult receives morphine sulfate gr $\frac{1}{6}$, how much morphine sulfate should a 6-month-old infant receive?

$$\frac{\text{infant's}}{\text{dose}} = \frac{\text{age in months}}{150 \text{ months}} \times \frac{\text{adult}}{\text{dose}}$$

$x = $ _____

Substitute values in Fried's Rule; complete calculations, and label your answer.

$$x = \frac{6 \text{ months}}{150 \text{ months}} \times \text{gr } \frac{1}{6}$$

$$x = \frac{1}{150} \times \text{gr } \frac{1}{1}$$

$x = $ gr $\dfrac{1}{150}$ is this infant's dose of morphine sulfate.

16. Doses based on the age of the child have definite limitations when the weight of the child varies greatly from "normal." <u>Clark's</u> <u>Rule</u> utilizes the relationship between body weight of the child and the weight of the average adult in estimating the drug dose. On the basis of weight (in this case for a child who weighs 60 pounds) the nurse may use _____ to estimate the dose for the child.

Clark's Rule

---

17. Clark's Rule states:

$$\frac{\text{child's}}{\text{dose}} = \frac{\text{weight in pounds}}{150 \text{ pounds (avg. adult)}} \times \frac{\text{adult}}{\text{dose}}$$

Substitute for the child in the preceding frame.

$$\frac{\text{child's}}{\text{dose}} = \frac{\rule{2cm}{0.4pt}}{150 \text{ pounds}} \times \frac{\text{adult}}{\text{dose}}$$

60 pounds

---

18. Working step by step together, try this problem:

Example:
An adult receives aspirin gr x. How many grains of aspirin would you give to a child weighing 45 pounds?

$$\frac{\text{child's}}{\text{dose}} = \frac{\text{weight in pounds}}{150 \text{ pounds}} \times \frac{\text{adult}}{\text{dose}}$$

$$x = \frac{?}{?} \times \text{gr } 10$$

(Substitute values.)

45 pounds
150 pounds

19. $x = \dfrac{45 \text{ pounds}}{150 \text{ pounds}} \times \text{gr } 10$

$x =$ _____

Finish solving the problem.

$x = \dfrac{45 \text{ pounds}}{150 \text{ pounds}} \times \text{gr } 10$

$x = \dfrac{3}{10} \times \text{gr } 10$

$x = \text{gr iii of aspirin would be given to this child.}$

---

20. Another example:

If an adult receives diphenhydramine hydrochloride (Benadryl) 50.0 mg, how much Benadryl would a child weighing 27 pounds receive?

$\dfrac{\text{child's}}{\text{dose}} = \dfrac{\text{weight in pounds}}{150 \text{ pounds}} \times \dfrac{\text{adult}}{\text{dose}}$

Substitute values in Clark's Rule and complete the problem.

$x = \dfrac{27 \text{ pounds}}{150 \text{ pounds}} \times 50.0 \text{ mg}$

$x = \dfrac{27}{3} \times 1.0 \text{ mg}$

$x = 9.0 \text{ mg of Benadryl would be given to this child.}$

---

21. The recommended dose of many pediatric drugs is frequently indicated as the amount of the drug to be administered for each kilogram of body weight. When the weight is known in pounds, you will need to convert to kilograms. Remember:

pounds ÷ 2.2 = kilograms.

Therefore, a 44-pound boy weighs

_____ kg.

20

22. Example:
Your client is a child weighing 54 pounds. Order: "Give acetaminophen 5 mg/kg q4h."

First: convert pounds to kilograms.

pounds ÷ 2.2 = kg

54 ÷ 2.2 = _____ kg   24.5 or 25

---

23. Second: this order is for acetaminophen 5 mg/kg; therefore, to obtain the dose, you will multiply:

mg × kg = dose

or

5 × 25 = _____ mg acetaminophen to be given every 4 hours.   125

---

24. Example:
The order reads "Dimenhydrinate (Dramamine) 1.25 mg/kg q6h." Your client's weight is 132 pounds.

First: pounds ÷ 2.2 = kg

132 ÷ 2.2 = _____ kg   60

---

25. Second: mg × kg = dose

1.25 × 60 = _____ mg Dramamine to be given every 6 hours.   75

Note: This method may be used for calculating drug dosage for adults as well as for infants and children.

26. Sometimes you will find the medication order written to cover a 24-hour period, and to be given in divided doses. Example: "600 mg/24 hours. Give in 6 equal doses."

To calculate the amount of the drug to be given at each time, you simply divide the amount of the drug to be given in 24 hours by the number of doses.

Total amount ÷ number of doses = amount/dose

In the example above:

600 mg ÷ 6 = _____ mg/dose

100

27. Example:
"Phenobarbital 2 mg/kg/24 hours. Give in 4 equal doses." The client's weight is 80 pounds.

Pounds ÷ 2.2 = kg

80 ÷ 2.2 = _____ kg

36

28. mg × kg = amount

2 × 36 = _____ mg/24 hours

72

29. 72 mg ÷ 4 doses = _____ mg of phenobarbital to be given four times in 24 hours.

18

30. Note: Another commonly used method to convert the dose per kilogram to dose per pound is to divide the given dose by 2.2 and then multiply by the weight in pounds.

Amount/kg ÷ 2.2 = the amount of drug given per pound of body weight.

Example:
If the order is for 50 mg/kg body weight for a child of 22 pounds, how many mg will be given?

Amt./kg ÷ 2.2 = Amt./pound

50 ÷ 2.2 = _____ mg/pound

22.7 or 23

31. Then:
Multiply mg/pound by the number of pounds body weight to determine the amount of drug for this child.

mg/pound × pounds = amount of drug.

23 × 22 = _____ mg drug

506 or 500

32. Try another problem:
"Give aminophylline 5 mg/kg stat." The client's weight is 100 pounds.

First: Amt./kg ÷ 2.2 = Amt./pound

5 ÷ 2.2 = _____ mg/pound

2.27

33. Then:
Total amt. = mg/pound × pounds

Total amt. = 2.27 × 100

x = _____ mg

227

On page 119 are some practice problems. Determine which rule to use, then work the problem.

PRACTICE PROBLEMS

MEDICATIONS FOR INFANTS AND CHILDREN

(ANSWERS ON PAGES 120–123)

---

1. If an adult receives tetracycline 250.0 mg every 6 hours, how much tetracycline would a child of 8 years receive every 6 hours?

2. What is the dosage of oxytetracycline (Terramycin) for a child weighing 30 pounds if an adult is receiving Terramycin 100.0 mg?

3. An adult receives 300,000 units of penicillin twice a day. How much penicillin would be a reasonable dosage for a 10-month-old infant to receive twice a day?

4. Order: "Give chloral hydrate p.o. 25 mg/kg stat." The weight of the client is 40 pounds.

5. An adult receives atropine sulfate gr $\frac{1}{150}$. How much atropine sulfate would a child weighing 90 pounds receive?

6. What would be a reasonable dosage of penicillin for a 3-year-old child if an adult is receiving penicillin 300,000 units twice a day?

7. Order: "Give aspirin 65 mg/kg/24 hours. (R) Divide into 6 equal doses." The weight of the client is 64 pounds.

8. What is the dosage of pentobarbital (Nembutal) for a 5-month-old infant if the adult dosage is 90.0 mg?

9. Order: "Give meperidine (Demerol) 1 mg/kg 1M stat." The client's weight is 22 pounds.

10. An average adult dose of atropine sulfate is gr $\frac{1}{150}$. How much atropine sulfate would you give to a 6-year-old child?

11. If an adult is receiving sulfisoxazole (Gantrisin) 0.5 g, how much Gantrisin would an infant of 6 months receive?

12. An adult is receiving 300,000 units of penicillin twice a day. How much penicillin would a child weighing 75 pounds receive twice a day?

ANSWERS TO PROBLEMS ON PAGE 119

MEDICATIONS FOR INFANTS AND CHILDREN

---

1. YOUNG'S RULE

$$\text{Child's dose} = \frac{\text{age (in years)}}{\text{age (in years)} + 12} \times \text{adult dose}$$

$$x = \frac{8 \text{ years}}{8 \text{ years} + 12} \times 250.0 \text{ mg}$$

$$x = \frac{8}{20} \times 250.0 \text{ mg}$$

$$x = \frac{2}{5} \times 250.0 \text{ mg}$$

$$x = \frac{2}{1} \times 50.0 \text{ mg}$$

$x = 100.0$ mg of tetracycline is this child's dose.

2. CLARK'S RULE

$$\text{Child's dose} = \frac{\text{weight in pounds}}{150 \text{ pounds}} \times \text{adult dose}$$

$$x = \frac{30 \text{ pounds}}{150 \text{ pounds}} \times 100.0 \text{ mg}$$

$$x = \frac{1}{5} \times 100.0 \text{ mg}$$

$x = 20.0$ mg Terramycin would be this child's dose.

3. FRIED'S RULE

$$\text{Infant's dose} = \frac{\text{age in months}}{150 \text{ months}} \times \text{adult dose}$$

$$x = \frac{10 \text{ months}}{150 \text{ months}} \times 300,000 \text{ U}$$

$$x = \frac{1}{15} \times 300,000 \text{ U}$$

$x = 20,000$ units of penicillin would be this infant's dose.

4. BODY WEIGHT

$kg = 40 \div 2.2$

$x = 18$

25 mg $\times$ 18 kg = 450 mg chloral hydrate to be given stat.

5. BODY WEIGHT

$\text{Child's dose} = \dfrac{\text{weight in pounds}}{150 \text{ pounds}} \times \text{adult dose}$

$x = \dfrac{90 \cancel{\text{ pounds}}}{150 \cancel{\text{ pounds}}} \times \text{gr } \dfrac{1}{150}$

$x = \dfrac{3}{5} \times \text{gr } \dfrac{1}{150}$

$x = \dfrac{1}{5} \times \text{gr } \dfrac{1}{50}$

$x = \text{gr } \dfrac{1}{250}$ of atropine sulfate would be this child's dose.

6. YOUNG'S RULE

$\text{Child's dose} = \dfrac{\text{age (in years)}}{\text{age (in years)} + 12} \times \text{adult dose}$

$x = \dfrac{3 \cancel{\text{ years}}}{3 \cancel{\text{ years}} + 12} \times 300{,}000 \text{ U}$

$x = \dfrac{3}{15} \times 300{,}000 \text{ U}$

$x = \dfrac{1}{5} \times 300{,}000 \text{ U}$

$x = 60{,}000 \text{ U}$ of penicillin would be a reasonable child's dose.

7. BODY WEIGHT

$kg = 64 \div 2.2$

$x = 29$

65 mg $\times$ 29 kg $\div$ 1,885 mg/24 hours

1,885 mg $\div$ 6 doses = 314 mg of aspirin/dose.

8. FRIED'S RULE

$$\text{Infant's dose} = \frac{\text{age in months}}{150 \text{ months}} \times \text{adult dose}$$

$$x = \frac{5 \text{ months}}{150 \text{ months}} \times 90.0 \text{ mg}$$

$$x = \frac{1}{30} \times 90.0 \text{ mg}$$

x = 3.0 mg of Nembutal is this infant's dose.

9. BODY WEIGHT

$$\text{kg} = 22 \div 2.2$$

$$x = 10$$

1 mg $\times$ 10 kg = 10 mg Demerol to be given IM stat.

10. YOUNG'S RULE

$$\text{Child's dose} = \frac{\text{age (in years)}}{\text{age (in years)} + 12} \times \text{adult dose}$$

$$x = \frac{6 \text{ years}}{6 \text{ years} + 12} \times \text{gr} \frac{1}{150}$$

$$x = \frac{6}{18} \times \text{gr} \frac{1}{150}$$

$$x = \frac{1}{3} \times \text{gr} \frac{1}{150}$$

x = gr $\frac{1}{450}$ of atropine sulfate is this child's dose.

11. YOUNG'S RULE

$$\text{Infant's dose} = \frac{\text{age in months}}{150 \text{ months}} \times \text{adult dose}$$

$$x = \frac{6 \text{ months}}{150 \text{ months}} \times 0.5 \text{ g}$$

$$x = \frac{1}{25} \times 0.5 \text{ g}$$

x = 0.02 g or 20.0 mg of Gantrisin would be the infant dose.

12. CLARK'S RULE

Child's dose $= \dfrac{\text{weight in pounds}}{150 \text{ pounds}} \times$ adult dose

$x = \dfrac{75 \text{ pounds}}{150 \text{ pounds}} \times 300{,}000 \text{ U}$

$x = \dfrac{1}{2} \times 300{,}000 \text{ U}$

$x = 150{,}000$ units of penicillin would be given to this child twice a day.

COMPREHENSIVE EXAMINATION

(ANSWERS ON PAGE 140)

Directions: Place the correct letter in the space provided.

1. 60.0 kg = ? g

    a. 0.006 g

    b. 0.06 g

    c. 600.0 g

    d. 6,000.0 g

    e. 60,000.0 g   **1.** _____

2. 75.0 mg = ? g

    a. 7,500.0 g

    b. 750.0 g

    c. 0.75 g

    d. 0.075 g

    e. 0.0075 g   **2.** _____

3. 25.0 ml = ? cc

    a. 2.5 cc

    b. 25.0 cc

    c. 250.0 cc

    d. 500.0 cc

    e. 2,500.0 cc   **3.** _____

4. 55.0 liters = _?_ ml

    a. 0.055 ml

    b. 0.05 ml

    c. 0.5 ml

    d. 5,500.0 ml

    e. 55,000.0 ml   **4.** _____

5. 25.4 cm = _____?_____ inch(es)

    a. 1 inch

    b. 5 inches

    c. 10 inches

    d. 12 inches

    e. 15 inches   **5.** _____

6. 12 inches = _____?_____ cm

    a. 25 cm

    b. 28 cm

    c. 30.5 cm

    d. 31.2 cm

    e. 36 cm   **6.** _____

7. 32°C = _____?_____°F

    a. 86.2°F

    b. 87.6°F

    c. 89.6°F

    d. 95°F

    e. 98.6°F   **7.** _____

8. 100°F = _____?_____°C

    a. 34°C

    b. 36.2°C

    c. 37°C

    d. 37.8°C

    e. 39°C   **8.** _____

9. In the apothecaries' system, fifteen and one-half grains is written as

   a. $15\frac{1}{2}$ grains

   b. grains $15\frac{1}{2}$

   c. xv $\frac{1}{2}$ grains

   d. grains xvss

   e. none of the above   9. _____

10. drams (ʒ) vi = minims (M.) _?_

   a. 40 M.

   b. 120 M.

   c. 230 M.

   d. 360 M.

   e. 400 M.   10. _____

11. ounces (ʒ) 8 = drams _?_

   a. 24 drams

   b. 36 drams

   c. 48 drams

   d. 52 drams

   e. 64 drams   11. _____

12. ounces 48 = pints _?_

   a. 2 pints

   b. 3 pints

   c. 4 pints

   d. 6 pints

   e. 7 pints   12. _____

13. quarts 10 = pints _?_

   a. 5 pints

   b. 15 pints

   c. 20 pints

   d. 25 pints

   e. 30 pints   13. _____

14. 240 drops = _?_ teaspoonful(s)

    a. 1 teaspoonful

    b. 2 teaspoonfuls

    c. 3 teaspoonfuls

    d. 4 teaspoonfuls

    e. 5 teaspoonfuls

14. _____

15. 5 tablespoonfuls = _?_ teaspoonfuls

    a. 10 teaspoonfuls

    b. 15 teaspoonfuls

    c. 20 teaspoonfuls

    d. 25 teaspoonfuls

    e. 30 teaspoonfuls

15. _____

16. 3 ounces = _?_ tablespoonfuls

    a. 2 tablespoonfuls

    b. 4 tablespoonfuls

    c. 6 tablespoonfuls

    d. 8 tablespoonfuls

    e. 10 tablespoonfuls

16. _____

17. 5.0 g = gr _?_

    a. gr 15

    b. gr 30

    c. gr 45

    d. gr 60

    e. gr 75

17. _____

18. gr viiss = _?_ g

    a. 0.025 g

    b. 0.5 g

    c. 0.75 g

    d. 1.0 g

    e. 2.5 g

18. _____

19. 180.0 g = ounces (oz.) _?_

   a. 6 oz.

   b. 10 oz.

   c. 250 oz.

   d. 540 oz.

   e. 5,400 oz.   **19.** _____

20. ℥xxx = _?_ cc

   a. 90 cc

   b. 260 cc

   c. 500 cc

   d. 750 cc

   e. 900 cc   **20.** _____

21. 4.2 cc = M. _?_

   a. 23 M.

   b. 40 M.

   c. 48 M.

   d. 60 M.

   e. 63 M.   **21.** _____

22. 150 pounds = _?_ kg

   a. 90 kg

   b. 149.6 kg

   c. 76 kg

   d. 68 kg

   e. 40 kg   **22.** _____

23. 21 kg = _____?_____ pounds

   a. 40 pounds

   b. 42 pounds

   c. 45.8 pounds

   d. 46.2 pounds

   e. 47 pounds   **23.** _____

24. You are to administer codeine sulfate gr ss. The tablets you have are labeled codeine sulfate 30.0 mg. How many tablet(s) will you administer?

a. $\frac{1}{2}$ tablet

b. 1 tablet

c. $1\frac{1}{2}$ tablets

d. 2 tablets

e. $2\frac{1}{2}$ tablets   **24.** _____

25. You are to administer Gantrisin 1.0 g. The tablets you have are labeled Gantrisin 0.5 g. How many tablet(s) will you administer?

a. $\frac{1}{2}$ tablet

b. 1 tablet

c. $1\frac{1}{2}$ tablets

d. 2 tablets

e. $2\frac{1}{2}$ tablets   **25.** _____

26. You are to administer phenobarbital 90.0 mg. The tablets you have are labeled phenobarbital gr ss. How many tablet(s) will you administer?

a. 1 tablet

b. 2 tablets

c. 3 tablets

d. 4 tablets

e. 5 tablets   **26.** _____

27. You have an oral medication bottle labeled "Elixir of Donnatol ʒi = gr xv." Your doctor ordered you to take gr xxx. How many teaspoonful(s) will you take?

a. $\frac{1}{2}$ teaspoonful

b. 1 teaspoonful

c. 2 teaspoonfuls

d. 3 teaspoonfuls

e. $3\frac{1}{2}$ teaspoonfuls   **27.** _____

130

28. You have a bottle labeled "Elixir of phenobarbital gr xv/cc." You are to administer 0.5 g orally. How many cc do you prepare?

a. 0.5 cc

b. 1 cc

c. 2 cc

d. 3 cc

e. 3.5 cc

28. _____

29. You are to give acetysalicylic acid gr x. You have acetysalicylic acid tablets gr iiss. How many tablet(s) do you need?

a. 0.25 tablet

b. 1.5 tablets

c. 2.25 tablets

d. 3.0 tablets

e. 4.0 tablets

29. _____

30. You are to give sulfasuxidine 2.0 g. The tablets you have are labeled sulfasuxidine gr viiss. How many tablet(s) will you give?

a. 0.25 tablet

b. 1.0 tablet

c. 2.25 tablets

d. 3.0 tablets

e. 4.0 tablets

30. _____

31. You are to give A.S.A. gr v. The tablets you have are labeled A.S.A. 0.3 g. How many tablet(s) will you give?

a. $\frac{1}{2}$ tablet

b. 1 tablet

c. $1\frac{1}{2}$ tablets

d. 2 tablets

e. 5 tablets

31. _____

32. You are to give Milk of Magnesia ℥i. How many cc is this?

    a. 10 cc

    b. 15 cc

    c. 20 cc

    d. 25 cc

    e. 30 cc   **32.** _____

33. You are to drink 1,000 cc of water in 8 hours. How many quarts (qt.) would this be?

    a. $\frac{1}{2}$ qt.

    b. 1 qt.

    c. $1\frac{1}{2}$ qt.

    d. 2 qt.

    e. $2\frac{1}{2}$ qt.   **33.** _____

34. You are to administer cascara ʒi. How many teaspoonful(s) would this be?

    a. $\frac{1}{2}$ teaspoonful

    b. 1 teaspoonful

    c. $1\frac{1}{2}$ teaspoonfuls

    d. 2 teaspoonfuls

    e. $2\frac{1}{2}$ teaspoonfuls   **34.** _____

35. You are to give digitalis leaf gr iss. The tablets you have are labeled 60 mg. How many tablet(s) will you give?

    a. $\frac{1}{2}$ tablet

    b. 1 tablet

    c. $1\frac{1}{2}$ tablets

    d. 2 tablets

    e. $2\frac{1}{2}$ tablets   **35.** _____

36. You are to administer penicillin 750,000 units intramuscularly. The bottle of penicillin is labeled 300,000 units/cc. How many cc will you administer?

   a. 0.4 cc

   b. 0.8 cc

   c. 1.5 cc

   d. 2.5 cc

   e. 3.5 cc   **36.** _____

37. You have Ancef containing 500.0 mg in 1.0 cc. You are to give 400.0 mg. How much solution will you give?

   a. 0.2 cc

   b. 0.5 cc

   c. 0.8 cc

   d. 1.25 cc

   e. 1.55 cc   **37.** _____

38. You have a solution of cortisone acetate 25.0 mg in 1.0 cc. You are to give 60.0 mg. How much solution will you give?

   a. 0.4 cc

   b. 0.8 cc

   c. 1.8 cc

   d. 2.4 cc

   e. 3.2 cc   **38.** _____

39. You are to give 50 units of regular insulin. You have on hand a bottle labeled: "Regular insulin U-100" and a 3-ml hypodermic syringe. How much solution would you give?

   a. 0.2 cc

   b. 0.5 cc

   c. 1.2 cc

   d. 1.5 cc

   e. 2.0 cc   **39.** _____

40. You are to give cephalothin sodium gr viiss. You have a vial labeled: "Cephalothin sodium 0.5 g in 2.0 cc." How much of this solution would you give?

    a. 0.2 cc

    b. 0.5 cc

    c. 1.2 cc

    d. 1.5 cc

    e. 2.0 cc   **40.** _____

41. What type of syringe would you use for the injection described in problem 40?

    a. tuberculin

    b. 3-ml hypodermic

    c. 5-ml hypodermic

    d. 10-ml hypodermic

    e. 30-ml hypodermic   **41.** _____

42. You are to give 100,000 units of sodium penicillin G from a multi-dose vial labeled: "Sodium penicillin G, 1,000,000 units per 10.0 cc." How many cc will you need to use?

    a. 1.0 cc

    b. 2.0 cc

    c. 5.0 cc

    d. 7.0 cc

    e. 10.0 cc   **42.** _____

43. You are to give atropine sulfate 0.3 mg. You have a bottle labeled: "Atropine sulfate gr $\frac{1}{150}$ per cc." How much solution do you need to use?

    a. 0.5 cc

    b. 0.75 cc

    c. 1.0 cc

    d. 1.5 cc

    e. 1.75 cc   **43.** _____

44. What type of syringe would you use for the injection described in problem 43?

a. tuberculin

b. insulin

c. 3-ml hypodermic

d. 5-ml hypodermic

e. 10-ml hypodermic   44. _____

45. You are to give chlorpromazine 0.075 g from a bottle labeled: "Chlorpromazine 25.0 mg per ml." How much solution will you use?

a. 1.5 ml

b. 2.0 ml

c. 3.0 ml

d. 3.5 ml

e. 4.0 ml   45. _____

46. You are to give atropine sulfate gr $\frac{1}{300}$. You have a bottle of solution labeled: "Atropine sulfate 0.4 mg per cc." How much solution will you use?

a. 0.5 cc

b. 1.0 cc

c. 1.5 cc

d. 2.0 cc

e. 2.5 cc   46. _____

47. You are to give 600,000 units of penicillin. You have a bottle labeled: "Penicillin 3,000,000 units per 10.0 cc." How much solution will you use?

a. 0.5 cc

b. 1.2 cc

c. 1.5 cc

d. 2.0 cc

e. 2.5 cc   47. _____

48. You have a vial containing 500 units of a drug in dry form. How much diluent will you use to prepare a solution containing 125 units of drug per cc?

a. 0.25 cc

b. 1.0 cc

c. 2.5 cc

d. 4.0 cc

e. 10.0 cc   48. _____

49. A vial of potassium penicillin G contains 3,000,000 units of the dry drug. How much diluent will be needed to make a solution that contains 400,000 units of this drug per cc?

a. 0.25 cc

b. 2.5 cc

c. 5.0 cc

d. 6.5 cc

e. 7.5 cc   49. _____

50. You have a vial containing 25.0 mg of a drug in dry form. How much diluent will you use to prepare a solution containing 2.0 mg of drug per cc?

a. 5.0 cc

b. 7.5 cc

c. 10.0 cc

d. 12.5 cc

e. 15.0 cc   50. _____

51. You are at home and need to prepare 8 oz. of a normal saline solution (0.9% strength). How many teaspoonful(s) of table salt will you add to 8 oz. of hot water?

a. $\frac{1}{2}$ teaspoonful

b. 1 teaspoonful

c. 2 teaspoonfuls

d. $2\frac{1}{2}$ teaspoonfuls

e. 3 teaspoonfuls   51. _____

52. You are to prepare 1,000.0 cc of 1:5,000 solution of potassium permanganate. You have a stock solution labeled potassium permanganate 1:1,000. How many cc of this stock solution do you need?

a. 100.0 cc

b. 200.0 cc.

c. 300.0 cc

d. 400.0 cc

e. 500.0 cc   **52.** _____

53. How many cc of diluent do you need to add to the stock solution in problem 52 in order to prepare the 1,000.0 cc of 1:5,000 potassium permanganate solution?

a. 900.0 cc

b. 800.0 cc

c. 700.0 cc

d. 600.0 cc

e. 500.0 cc   **53.** _____

54. If an adult received Demerol 75.0 mg, what would you consider an appropriate dose of Demerol for an infant 10 months old?

a. 3.5 mg

b. 5.0 mg

c. 7.5 mg

d. 25.0 mg

e. 34.0 mg   **54.** _____

55. An adult is receiving tetracycline 250.0 mg, 4 times a day. Which of the following dosages would be considered a safe single dose for a child weighing 30 pounds?

a. 5.0 mg

b. 8.0 mg

c. 30.0 mg

d. 50.0 mg

e. 80.0 mg   **55.** _____

56. How much aspirin would you consider a safe dosage for a child of 4 years if an adult received aspirin gr x?

    a. gr iiss

    b. gr iii

    c. gr v

    d. gr viii

    e. gr x   **56.** _____

57. Order: "Theophylline 3 mg/pound q6h." The order is written for a child who weighs 36 pounds. Every 6 hours, you will give _____ mg theophylline.

    a. 237 mg

    b. 48 mg

    c. 75 mg

    d. 108 mg

    e. 14 mg   **57.** _____

58. Give 500 cc packed cells over a period of 4 hours. Your blood set delivers 10 drops/cc. What is the flow rate?

    a. 10 drops/min.

    b. 15 drops/min.

    c. 20 drops/min.

    d. 25 drops/min.

    e. 40 drops/min.   **58.** _____

59. Order: "100 cc lactated Ringer's solution in 8 hours." Using a Pedi-set, the flow rate will be _____ microdrops/min.

    a. 8 microdrops/min.

    b. 10 microdrops/min.

    c. 12 microdrops/min.

    d. 14 microdrops/min.

    e. 30 microdrops/min.   **59.** _____

60. Order: "1,000 cc D$_5$W to run at a rate of 125 cc per hour." What is the flow rate if the set delivers 15 gtt/cc?

    a. 3.1 gtt/min.

    b. 6.5 gtt/min.

    c. 31 gtt/min.

    d. 38 gtt/min.

    e. 45 gtt/min.   **60.** _____

61. Order "3,000 cc D$_5$W over 24 hours." What is the flow rate if the drop factor is 10 gtt/cc?

    a. 15 gtt/min.

    b. 17 gtt/min.

    c. 21 gtt/min.

    d. 25 gtt/min.

    e. 30 gtt/min.   **61.** _____

62. Order "Aminophylline 50 mg/hr. The solution is 200 mg of aminophylline in 250 ml $\frac{1}{2}$ NSS." How many ml per hour are to be infused?

    a. 10 ml/hr

    b. 25.5 ml/hr

    c. 31 ml/hr

    d. 62.5 ml/hr

    e. 100 ml/hr   **62.** _____

63. Order: "IV 1,000 cc PSS with 40,000 units of heparin to infuse at 75 ml/hr." What is the dose of heparin delivered every hour?

    a. 1,000 units

    b. 2,000 units

    c. 3,000 units

    d. 4,000 units

    e. 5,000 units   **63.** _____

ANSWERS TO COMPREHENSIVE EXAM

1. e	**22.** d	**43.** b
2. d	**23.** d	**44.** a
3. b	**24.** b	**45.** c
4. e	**25.** d	**46.** a
5. c	**26.** c	**47.** d
6. c	**27.** c	**48.** d
7. c	**28.** a	**49.** e
8. d	**29.** e	**50.** d
9. d	**30.** e	**51.** a
10. d	**31.** b	**52.** b
11. e	**32.** e	**53.** b
12. b	**33.** b	**54.** b
13. c	**34.** b	**55.** d
14. d	**35.** c	**56.** a
15. b	**36.** d	**57.** d
16. c	**37.** c	**58.** c
17. e	**38.** d	**59.** c
18. b	**39.** b	**60.** c
19. a	**40.** e	**61.** c
20. e	**41.** b	**62.** d
21. e	**42.** a	**63.** c